The Menopause Thyroid Solution

Also by MARY J. SHOMON

The
MENOPAUSE
THYROID SOLUTION

* *

Overcome Menopause
by Solving Your Hidden
Thyroid Problems

* *

Mary J. Shomon

HARPER

NEW YORK · LONDON · TORONTO · SYDNEY

HARPER

HarperCollins books may be purchased for educational, business, or sales promotional use. For information, please write: Special Markets Department, HarperCollins Publishers, 10 East 53rd Street, New York, NY 10022.

FIRST EDITION

Designed by Janet M. Evans

Library of Congress Cataloging-in-Publication Data
Shomon, Mary J.
    The menopause thyroid solution : overcome menopause by solving your hidden thyroid problems / Mary J. Shomon. — 1st ed.
        p. cm.
Includes bibliographical references.
    ISBN 978-0-06-158264-6
    1. Menopause. 2. Thyroid hormones—Metabolism. 3. Thyroid gland—Diseases—Diagnosis. I. Title.
    RG186.S6656 2009
    618.1'75—dc22

2008048299

09 10 11 12 13   OV/RRD   10 9 8 7 6 5 4 3 2 1

There is no more creative
force in the world than
the menopausal woman
with zest.
—Margaret Mead

All adventures, especially
into new territory, are scary.
—Sally Ride

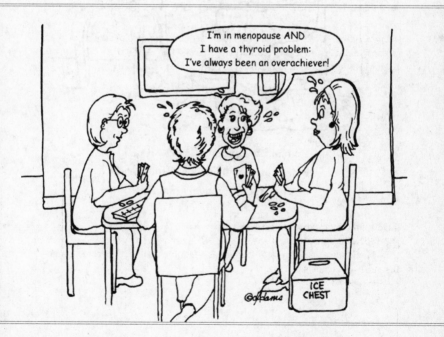

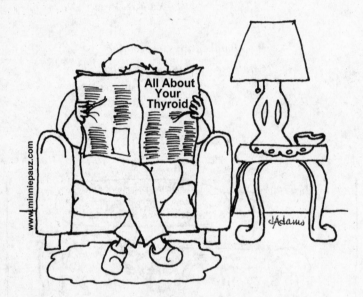

Hmmm...the symptoms are fatique,
weight gain, and memory problems.
That sounds vaguely familiar.

acknowledgments

This book wouldn't be possible without my family, Jon, Julia, and Danny Mathis, who have been so patient, yet quick with the hugs and support, when I'm knee deep into writing. I am always grateful for the friendship of my "soul sister" Jeannie Yamine, who is always ready to listen, brainstorm, and cheer me on. Thanks also to the rest of the family—especially my father, Dan Shomon Sr.; brother, Dan Shomon Jr.; in-laws, Rus and Barb Mathis; and cousins Ellen Blaze and Joan Kelleher—for their support. And to my mother, Pat, thanks for always being with me in spirit.

Many thanks to HarperCollins and Jessica Deputato, for her tremendous assistance and enthusiasm for this book. I am always grateful to be represented by a phenomenal agent and friend, Carol Mann of the Carol Mann Agency. I don't want to miss a chance for a final thank you to my editor for the last ten years, Sarah Durand. My previous books are better for having been edited by Sarah.

I could not have finished this book without the research/writing help of Cynthia Austin and Leslie Blumenberg and the wonderful babysitting of Rosario Quintanilla and Elizabeth Mensah Engmann.

I must thank the experts who keep me healthy and happy: Kate Lemmerman, MD, Jan Nicholson, and Scott Kwiatkowski, DO. Also, thanks to my New York colleagues Aracely Brown at the New York

Open Center and Robyn Hartman of the Women's Wellness Society and to my New York About.com editorial team of Joy Walsh Victory, Kate Grossman, Stacey Felsen, and Kristin Kane.

Thanks to my dearest friends, who make this world a better place: Mohammed Antabli and Franca Fiabane, Michael Phillips, Gen Piturro and Demo DeMartile, Julia Schopick, Richard Moss, Jane and Joe Frank, Kathlin Smith and Bernie Van Leer, Cynthia Austin, Laura Horton, Kim Conley, and the "Momfriends."

Thanks also go to the many thyroid patients who generously contributed their personal stories for the book, including support group guru Stefanie Rotsaert, and to my unofficial news bureau: Kim Carmichael Cox, Sherry Leu, and Micki Jacobs, for making sure I don't miss any of the latest news.

Much gratitude goes to the practitioners and professionals who generously shared their time, information, resources, and insights for this book or helped facilitate my information-gathering process. They include David Brownstein, MD; Adrienne Clamp, MD, DABMA; Annemarie Colbin, PhD; Jocelyne Eberstein, LAc, DOM; Laura Fredrick of McKinney Advertising & Public Relations; Ann Louise Gittleman, PhD, CNS; Gayle Green; Stephen Gurgevich, PhD; Joy Gurgevich; Charles Hakala and Hakala Labs/Research; Harriet Hall, MD; Donna Hurlock, MD; Irma Jennings; Risa Kagan, MD, FACOG; Scott Kwiatkowski, DO; Tieraona Low Dog, MD; Eileen Mackison; Martin Mulders, MD; Viana Muller, PhD; the North American Menopause Society; Tara Parker-Pope; Walter Pierpaoli, MD; Jerilynn Prior, MD, FRCPC; Uzzi Reiss, MD; Teri Robert, PhD; Molly Roberts, MD; Marie Savard, MD; Karilee Shames, RN, PhD; Richard Shames, MD; Jan Shifren, MD; Kim Switnicki, ACC, ECPC; Teresa Tapp and Kitty Etherly of T-Tapp; Jacob Teitelbaum, MD; and David Zava and ZRT Laboratories. Thanks also to Dee Adams for the amazing cartoons and her unfailing sense of humor.

contents

chapter 1

Menopause and Thyroid
AN INTRODUCTION

> After thirty, a body has a mind of its own.
>
> —*Bette Midler*

As a woman born in 1961, I'm lucky to be part of the generation of baby boomers who are likely to live well into our seventies or eighties. All of us want to get to that age feeling as healthy and energetic as possible. After all, we're the generation that has come up with the popular mantras "Fifty is the new forty," "Sixty is the new fifty," and so on.

So here we are, living longer than ever. For many of us, our forties and fifties are a time when we are hitting our professional stride, our children are growing up and leaving home, and we can turn our attention to taking care of ourselves.

Why is it that just when you're coming into your own, it seems as if your body is falling apart?

You start gaining weight and feeling bloated. You find it harder to remember things and nearly impossible to concentrate. You notice your cholesterol level is going up, even though you haven't changed your diet. Your moods shift quickly: sometimes you're anxious; other times you feel blue and depressed. You're exhausted, but at bedtime, you feel restless and find it hard to sleep. You feel hot, then cold—the temperature is never right. Every time you shampoo or run a brush through your hair, a handful of hair comes out. Periods? They're erratic and unpredictable, and when they do come, they're sometimes so heavy you can't even leave the house. And sex? What's that?

So you jump to what seems like a logical conclusion: "Menopause!" (And if you don't assume it, your doctor will happily assume it for you.)

By *menopause*, I'm actually taking some liberties with the term and talking about the whole perimenopause-into-menopause transition, a process that can sometimes take as long as eight to ten years. Many people use the terms *menopause* and *perimenopause* interchangeably to refer to the entire transition process. In this book, I actually do this too at times, even in the title, because, let's face it, we're more likely to connect hot flashes, night sweats, erratic periods, and such with the idea of menopause. But apparently, 90 percent of us go through four to eight years of fluctuating hormones, erratic periods, and then, finally, that last menstrual period. Officially, the entire process is known as perimenopause or, less commonly, "premenopause." Officially, menopause is confirmed when it's been a year since your last period. After that last period, it's "postmenopause."

If you say "I'm going through menopause," and you are still having periods, then you are actually going through perimenopause. If you've stopped having periods for at least a year, you are technically postmenopausal.

You may not realize that by the time you are one year past your last menstrual period (again, menopause) your symptoms usually have improved and often have disappeared. That's because it's not the lack of hormones that causes symptoms in most women. It's actually the up-and-down fluctuations in hormones, as well as imbalances in the ratio of hormones, that take place in the months and years before that last period that cause the most troublesome symptoms.

Anyway, back to the symptoms. You start feeling exhausted, gain weight, become overheated, lose your hair, develop a low sex drive, and notice assorted aches and pains, so you assume you're in menopause. And off you go, to try to deal with it all.

You may start drinking soy smoothies, munching on soy burgers and edamame, and popping every menopause-manipulating herb available, from black cohosh to dong quai to chasteberry. Or you smear yourself with wild yam cream. Or you end up taking out a second mortgage to pay for complicated, compounded bioidentical hormone regimens. Or you head to the doctor, who sends you off with Premarin or Prempro—the prescription conjugated estrogen drugs made from horse urine—then every time you take a pill, you're worried that you're increasing your risk for breast cancer or stroke.

And the saddest part of all? For some of you, *none of this will help.*

Why? Because it's missing the point.

You're forgetting what may be the most important hormone of all: thyroid hormone.

By age sixty, as many as half of all women have a slowdown in the thyroid, the master gland of metabolism and energy. And guess what the most common symptoms are? Fatigue, weight gain, depression, anxiety, menstrual irregularities, low sex drive, hair loss, and brain fog/memory problems.

So when you and your doctor assume that your symptoms are "hormonal," you may be partially right, but the critical hormone you're overlooking may be thyroid hormone.

The natural decline of estrogen and progesterone that occurs in women starting in our late thirties—and which is happening now to millions of American women—is one of the most common triggers of a thyroid slowdown. The shocker is that the millions of baby boomers who are in thyroid slowdown *are not even diagnosed.*

Instead, these women—and their doctors—are assuming they are menopausal. These women then spend thousands of dollars a year on appointments, pills, and potions to try to stave off menopausal symptoms and never get thyroid tests.

A near epidemic is being overlooked in this, an otherwise empowered, informed generation of women.

That's why we need a solution: *The Menopause Thyroid Solution*.

• • •

Why are baby boomer and menopausal women at such a risk for thyroid problems? There are actually several key reasons.

- First, thyroid problems are simply more prevalent as we age. Like many organs, the thyroid tends to slow down as we get older. So, as we age, we are generally at greater risk of developing thyroid problems.

- Second, busy baby boomer women frequently face a high degree of physical stress—improper diet, lack of exercise, not enough sleep, exposures to toxins—as well as emotional and life stresses. Chronic stress causes the adrenal glands to ramp up production of stress hormones. There are limited raw materials to produce hormones, and the body considers survival more important than thyroid function, so chronic stress shifts production away from making thyroid hormone and toward making stress hormones. Eventually, if you push the adrenals long enough, adrenal fatigue sets in, which puts even more strain on the thyroid.

- Third, hormone fluctuations during this period can affect the thyroid. When the ratio of estrogen to progesterone becomes imbalanced, even if both hormones are declining, a situation known as estrogen dominance can develop. Estrogen dominance can prevent thyroid hormone molecules from properly binding with receptors, making thyroid hormone unavailable to your cells, and leaves you functionally hypothyroid at the cellular level.

– Fourth, thyroid hormone has some chemical similarities to estrogen. The various receptor sites for thyroid, found throughout the body, can, therefore, be blocked by the presence of estrogen. Taking supplemental estrogen, as some women do when they are experiencing what they think are menopausal symptoms, can prevent thyroid hormone molecules from properly binding with the receptors, which makes the thyroid hormone unavailable to the cells.

– Finally, as progesterone levels drop, which is characteristic in perimenopause and menopause, thyroid hormone requirements typically increase. Sufficient progesterone is actually necessary to ensure adequate binding of T3 (triiodothyronine), the active thyroid hormone.

Thyroid problems also worsen perimenopausal/menopausal symptoms. This means that women who don't know they have a thyroid problem and go into this period of hormonal flux may suffer more than other women. Women who know they have a thyroid problem but who aren't being properly or effectively treated may also suffer more.

How do thyroid problems trigger or worsen perimenopausal/menopausal symptoms? There are four key ways.

– First, as noted, the thyroid slows as we age. As the thyroid becomes less functional, it is less able to perform its job of delivering energy to organs and glands. Reproductive organs like the ovaries are no exception.

– Second, when chronic stress causes a hormone shift toward adrenal/stress hormones and away from thyroid hormone, it also shifts away from reproductive hormone production. Over time, in addition to causing thyroid conditions, stress-triggered adrenal fatigue can cause reductions in estrogen and progesterone.

– Third, thyroid imbalances can disrupt the hormone production pathway. Thyroid hormone is essential to the process of converting cholesterol into pregnenolone, which is then converted into progesterone, DHEA (dehydroepiandrosterone), estrogen, and testosterone. So any deficiency of thyroid hormone can disrupt the entire hormone production process.

– Finally, anovulatory cycles (cycles where you don't ovulate) are more common in thyroid patients. These can contribute to a deficiency in progesterone, which can affect perimenopause.

If we have what some practitioners consider an epidemic of undiagnosed thyroid problems in American women, and these problems may be the cause of symptoms in a substantial number of women in perimenopause/menopause, why isn't it standard for women to get tested and treated?

The problem is that perimenopause/menopause is a confusing time. Because thyroid problems often develop in women at the same age as perimenopausal or menopausal symptoms, and they share many symptoms, it can be difficult to figure out the real problem.

Except for traditional hot flashes and night sweats that last a few minutes, vaginal/bladder problems, and sagging/tender breasts, the symptoms of perimenopause and menopause are *exactly* the same as the symptoms of a thyroid problem. Still, doctors—and women—are far more familiar with sex hormone imbalances than they are with thyroid problems.

Unfortunately, according to a survey conducted by the American Association of Clinical Endocrinologists, only one in four women who have discussed menopause with their physician actually receive a recommendation to be tested for thyroid disease. Doctors are assuming that perimenopause/menopause is the one and only issue at hand. Or, in some cases, there's an assumption that symptoms may be due to the stage in life. Says patient advocate and physician Marie Savard, MD:

> All too often doctors attribute these symptoms to stress and women becoming "empty nesters." I'll never forget my GYN textbook in medical school that described menopause symptoms of depression, fatigue, etc., and clearly said they were due to "empty nest syndrome" and not hormonal changes.

Thyroid testing is also not part of any standard screening, nor are thyroid tests part of most annual physicals—no matter what your age.

Another challenge to getting diagnosed is that it's difficult to find doctors who will listen to and explore our symptoms. We're a generation of women who are being faced with shorter than ever appointments with doctors and revolving-door HMOs.

It's also a challenge because there's sometimes the assumption that it's normal to not feel well as we age. Hormonal expert David Brownstein, MD, explains:

> Women need to be aware that if they are feeling tired, brain fogged, and not thinking clearly, these sorts of symptoms are not "a normal part of aging." You don't have to feel like all of a sudden you've aged fifteen years overnight. If that happens, something is wrong. And one of those things that frequently show up is thyroid problems. When they're rectified, you can feel back to normal. You don't have to feel like you're eighteen, but brainwise, you should feel as good. If you're not, that's something that needs to be brought forward. Investigating the thyroid at the time of hormonal change is appropriate.

Another challenge is that hormones are a big business. There's far more profit to be made in selling you Premarin and Prempro, bioidentical hormones, and herbal menopause remedies than in diagnosing and treating a thyroid condition. Take a look in any women's magazine, and count up the number of ads and articles about menopause treatments. Then look for ads and articles about thyroid treatments. You'll see what I mean.

Tieraona Low Dog, MD, says that medicine has made menopause an "estrogen deficiency disease." She says:

> There's a societal attitude promoting menopause as something to be treated because there's a huge business around menopause, and to sell a drug, you have to convince people that there's something they need to take it for.

According to research company Datamonitor, sales of hormone replacement drugs in the United States alone topped $2 billion in 2008. If you were to pay out of pocket, a typical monthly supply of thyroid medication costs from around $15 to $23. The least expensive combination estrogen/progesterone therapy, Premphase, will run you more than $60 a month. A brand name combination regimen of an estradiol patch like Climara plus Prometrium progesterone costs more than $150 a month. "Follow the money," as they say.

• • •

Could you be one of the millions of women suffering what you think are perimenopausal/menopausal symptoms but are actually dealing with an undiagnosed thyroid condition?

I know some of you are thinking, I'm not fat, so I can't have a thyroid problem. "Thyroid problem" has become secret code for comedians and advertisers who want to make fun of overweight, middle-aged women. It's true; some people with thyroid problems do struggle with extra weight. But there are plenty of thin thyroid patients out there, too.

In fact, there's no way to look at yourself in the mirror and rule out a thyroid condition. While many women simply don't know anything about the thyroid, some women have the idea that in addition to weight problems, thyroid patients must have an enlarged or lumpy neck (a goiter) or protruding eyeballs. Not so. Many thyroid patients have no visible signs at all. The only way to properly diagnose a thyroid problem is for your doctor to conduct a thorough thyroid exam and run the appropriate tests.

But there are some signs to look for that suggest it may be your thyroid.

First, if you are perimenopausal/menopausal, and your doctor has put you on estrogen or hormone therapy, and it's not working—or not working well enough—it could be your thyroid. An estimated one-third of the women who take estrogen therapy still experience symptoms, which are most often attributed to menopause but may be thyroid-related.

And, as noted, estrogen can actually block thyroid receptors, so if you have a thyroid condition that hasn't been diagnosed, you might actually feel worse after starting an estrogen drug.

Hormone expert Richard Shames, MD, explains:

What is classic for this group is that you can be told you're in "menopause"—and not knowing it's actually your thyroid, you take estrogen. That will help a few of your menopause symptoms, but everything else can be a little worse. You end up gaining weight and losing hair, but you chalk it up to menopause. Meanwhile, the estrogen has decreased your thyroid function even more.

Second, you need to work with a doctor who can help differentiate your symptoms. According to gynecologist and menopause expert Donna Hurlock, MD:

If you have an underlying thyroid problem, you can replace estrogen all day and all night and it won't improve until you improve the thyroid. And if you give estrogen to a woman, and her symptoms get worse, that's often a sign that it's the thyroid as well. I look at the symptoms. It seems in my experience that women who come in before fifty who have erratic periods are more often dealing with an underactive thyroid. If I see hair loss, that's usually a sign that it's thyroid and not menopause. If a woman has dry skin, then thyroid is more often a player than estrogen. Brain fog and fuzziness are more often thyroid than estrogen. And sex drive improves more with thyroid. Vaginal dryness? That is probably estrogen. I was taught that hot flashes are due to lack of estrogen, but that's not always true. Hot flashes and irregular menses can be thyroid. If a woman feels hot for twenty minutes and then it goes, that's often thyroid. If she's estrogen deficient, a woman should actually be hot to the touch. If a woman has ice cold hands but feels hot, that's often thyroid.

What can you do? After all, no one is going to institute mandatory thyroid testing for women over forty. Thyroid tests aren't part of a standard physical, and no one is going to make it standard practice to give thyroid tests to women with perimenopausal/menopausal symptoms.

The truth is, it's up to you.

The only way to find out if your thyroid is causing—or aggravating—your symptoms is to insist on getting tested, diagnosed, and treated. If you are a woman with perimenopausal/menopausal symptoms, you need to get your thyroid evaluated and treated right away—the *right* way.

There's a catch, of course. The only way it's going to happen may be for you to be your own advocate.

"But why isn't my doctor doing this?" you may ask. "It's like I have to be my own doctor!" And yes, it is unfair to think that you have to take responsibility, ask for tests that your doctor isn't suggesting, insist that they be properly interpreted, and push for proper treatment.

But let's get past what's fair and get to what's necessary. You owe it to yourself. Like me, you may be one of the millions of women whose health depends on your thyroid, and unresolved problems in this critical gland will wreak hormonal havoc. Let's look at the reality.

- Thyroid problems can send you into a far too early perimenopause—starting as early as age forty—and it can last for years. Doesn't that sound like fun?

- Thyroid problems can worsen any perimenopausal and postmenopausal symptoms. This means you multiply the intensity or discomfort of everything from erratic, heavy periods, to hot flashes, to dizziness, to heart palpitations. You could even end up with an unneeded hysterectomy.

- Thyroid problems can slow your metabolism and destabilize your blood sugar so much that it's not only impossible to lose weight, you actually gain weight— on fewer calories than everyone else. And where are you most likely to gain? Where else but your belly, of course.

- Thyroid problems can make you so depressed, stressed, or both, that you're prescribed antidepressants, antianxiety drugs, and tranquilizers, not to mention sleeping pills.

- Thyroid problems can impair your memory and make you so foggy-brained that you are needlessly worried you are developing Alzheimer's disease.

- Thyroid problems can raise your cholesterol and triglycerides to such dangerous levels that you must go on medication to protect your arteries and heart.

- Thyroid problems can elevate your blood pressure to levels that require prescription medications.

- Thyroid problems can make your hair fall out so quickly that you worry whether you're actually going to go bald. (Believe me, there are few things as demoralizing for a middle-aged woman as realizing she's losing her hair.)

- Thyroid problems can exhaust you to the extent that you have no energy for exercise, which affects fitness, weight, heart disease risk, and quality of life.

- Thyroid problems can wear down your immune system's effectiveness to the extent that you catch every infection you're exposed to and, once ill, are slower to recover.

- Thyroid problems can deplete your body's ability to cope with stress so much that you feel extremely tired yet wired most of the time and suffer anxiety and insomnia along with your fatigue.

If we want to truly take charge of our hormonal health, we need to pay close attention to the thyroid.

Most doctors aren't doing it.

The "menopause gurus" aren't doing it.

The people selling menopause remedies and medications aren't doing it.

The aging TV stars who are making money promoting hormone information (you know, these days you can get menopause advice from the former stars of *Charlie's Angels* and *Three's Company*) aren't doing it.

The media aren't doing it.

Even Oprah's not doing it, and she's hypothyroid and menopausal.

In the end, it's up to us.

We are part of a generation that believes in making a difference. Now we have a chance to find solutions, to do something that will help our hormonal health, metabolism, mental health, and nearly every facet of our well-being, well into old age.

In *The Menopause Thyroid Solution*, you are going to learn not only how to get your thyroid problems diagnosed and treated, but how to maintain "the balancing act": balancing the thyroid with the other hormones in the key reproductive and stress/adrenal hormone pathways.

Along the way, *The Menopause Thyroid Solution* will help you

- Know whether you are at extra risk of developing a thyroid condition.

- Recognize the common—and not so common—symptoms of thyroid problems and perimenopause/menopause.

- Learn how to get thyroid and hormonal imbalance problems properly diagnosed (it's often a challenge). You'll learn how to do this regardless of whether you have the best medical insurance in town or a barely so-so HMO, or even if you need to go the route of self-testing.

- Explore how best to treat your thyroid condition, including prescription medications, supplements, herbs, nutrition, and other approaches.

- Understand how to manage and address thyroid, reproductive/sex hormones (estrogen, progesterone, testosterone, etc.) and adrenal balance.

- Find out what and how to eat, what medications to consider, what supplements to take, and which mind–body approaches to practice, in order to balance your hormones.

- Improve your metabolism for more effective weight management or even weight loss.

As a woman, you're knowledgeable and empowered. You have access to more information than ever before, and you've always felt like you could change the world.

What better way to start than for each and every woman to enjoy the best possible hormonal health? Let's get started!

chapter 2

Could It Be Your
THYROID?

The heyday of woman's life is the shady side of fifty.
—Elizabeth Cady Stanton

Let's start by taking a look at the endocrine system, and the thyroid, and the risks and symptoms of thyroid disease.

The Endocrine System

First, it's important to understand that the thyroid and the reproductive system are all part of what's known as the endocrine system. The endocrine system is made up of organs, some of which are also known as glands, whose primary purpose is to release hormones. The major endocrine organs and glands in women, their location, and the key hormones they release are the

- Pineal gland, located in the brain, which releases melatonin

- Pituitary gland, located in the brain, which releases

adrenocorticotropic hormone (ACTH), thyroid-stimulating hormone (TSH), prolactin, growth hormone (GH), endorphins, follicle-stimulating hormone (FSH), and luteinizing hormone (LH)

- Thyroid gland, located in the neck, which releases primarily thyroxine (T4), triiodothyronine (T3), and calcitonin, but also diiodothyronine (T2) and monoiodothyronine (T1)

- Parathyroid glands, located next to the thyroid in the neck, which release parathyroid hormone (PTH)

- Thymus, located in the chest, which releases thymosins, hormones that help immune system cells function

- Adrenal glands, located over the kidneys, which release cortisol, adrenaline (epinephrine), noradrenaline (norepinephrine), dopamine, testosterone, androstenedione, and aldosterone

- Pancreas, located in the abdominal area, which releases insulin, glucagon, somatostatin, and pancreatic polypeptide

- Ovaries, located in the pelvic region, which release estrogens, progesterone, testosterone, dehydroepiandrosterone (DHEA), and inhibin

The hypothalamus, located in the brain, functions as part of both the endocrine system and the nervous system and acts as a link between them. The hypothalamus acts as the endocrine system's primary coordinator and command center, releasing hormones to help control the other glands' activities and coordinating the various glands and hormonal cycles. Another key role of the hypothalamus is as the starting point for the female menstrual cycle. The hypothalamus releases gonadotropin-releasing hormone (GnRH), which causes the pituitary to stimulate the ovaries to develop egg follicles and set the process into motion. The hypothalamus also releases thyrotropin-releasing hormone (TRH), growth hormone–releasing hormone (GHRH), corticotropin-releasing hormone (CRH), somatostatin, and dopamine.

Because the endocrine organs and glands operate in similar ways and are interconnected, they are viewed as one system.

In addition to the key endocrine organs and glands, other organs play a part in the endocrine system by releasing hormones. These include the stomach, which releases gastrin, ghrelin, neuropeptide Y, and secretin; the small intestine, which releases secretin and cholecystokinin; the heart, which releases atriopeptin; and the placenta, which releases human chorionic gonadotropin (HCG). Fat tissue itself can become like an endocrine gland, releasing leptin and estrogens.

The Thyroid and Thyroid Hormone

The thyroid is a small bow tie- or butterfly-shaped gland that normally weighs about an ounce. It is situated in the lower part of the neck, in front of the windpipe, and slightly behind and below the Adam's apple area. The two "wings" of the butterfly-shaped gland are known as the lobes of the thyroid, and the area connecting the two lobes is known as the isthmus.

The thyroid's most important purpose is to produce, store, and release two key thyroid hormones: triiodothyronine, abbreviated as T3, and thyroxine, abbreviated as T4. The 3 and the 4 refer to the number of iodine molecules attached to each hormone.

The thyroid is able to produce this hormone by absorbing iodine, an essential nutrient, from food, iodized salt, and supplements. Iodine is then combined with the amino acid tyrosine to produce T4 and T3. Of the thyroid hormone produced by a healthy thyroid gland, about 80 percent is T4, and 20 percent is T3. T3 is the biologically active hormone that is used by the cells and is several times stronger than T4. The body converts the inactive T4 to active T3 by removing one iodine molecule (known as T4-to-T3 conversion, or monodeiodination). This conversion of T4 to T3 can take place in the thyroid or other organs, including the hypothalamus, a part of the brain.

T4 and T3 exist in two forms: free/unbound and bound. Free or unbound T4 or T3 refers to that part that is biologically active, and the bound part is attached to the thyroxine-binding globulin (TBG) protein. When measured in the blood, the free or unbound T4 and T3 levels tend to give the most accurate picture of the actual thyroid hormone available for use by the body.

Once it gets to the cells, what does thyroid hormone do? The role of thyroid hormone is to control metabolism. That means, thyroid hormone controls the process by which oxygen and calories are converted to the energy your cells and organs need. Specifically, thyroid hormone helps

Cells convert oxygen and calories into energy

The heart pump properly and effectively

The nervous system function properly

The intestinal system properly digest and eliminate food

The brain function properly

Strengthen hair, nails, and skin

Process carbohydrates

In the proper functioning of muscles

In the proper functioning of the immune system

With sexual development and functioning

With respiration (breathing)

With normal bone growth

• • •

As you can see, the thyroid has an impact on every aspect of your health.

THE THYROID FEEDBACK LOOP

When the thyroid is working properly, it produces and secretes the amount of T4 and T3 your body needs to function. The thyroid works, however, as part of a bigger system—a feedback loop that includes the pituitary gland and the hypothalamus. Here's how the system works.

The hypothalamus monitors and reacts to a number of body functions, as well as environmental factors like heat, cold, and illness. When the hypothalamus senses that the body is facing a stressor, it produces TRH.

TRH is sent from the hypothalamus to the pituitary gland. The pituitary gland is stimulated to produce a substance called thyrotropin, better known as TSH. The pituitary gland is also monitoring the circulating levels of thyroid hormone in the body and releases (or stops releasing) TSH based on the thyroid hormone levels circulating in the blood.

Once released, TSH is sent to the thyroid gland, where it stimulates the thyroid to produce, store, and release more T3 and T4 thyroid hormones.

The released thyroid hormones move into the bloodstream, carried by a plasma protein known as TBG.

Now in the bloodstream, the thyroid hormone travels throughout the body to the various organs. Upon arriving at a particular tissue in the body, thyroid hormone interacts with receptors located inside the nuclei of the cells. Interaction of the hormone and the receptor will trigger a certain function, giving directions to that tissue regarding the rate at which it should operate.

When the hypothalamus senses that the need for increased thyroid hormone production has ended, it reduces production of TRH. The reduced production of TRH in turn causes the pituitary to decrease production of TSH, and the reduced TSH levels send the message to the gland itself to slow production of thyroid hormone.

Like the thermostat in your house set to a particular temperature, your body is set to maintain a certain level of circulating thyroid hormone. It is when disease or damage to the thyroid gland takes place, or the feedback process malfunctions, that we see thyroid problems developing.

THYROID CONDITIONS

Thyroid problems are widespread, and the European Thyroid Association estimates that more than 200 million people around the world have thyroid disease. The most extensive problems are seen in areas covered in the past by glaciers, where there is not enough iodine in the soil and the crops grown in that soil. (Iodine is necessary for proper thyroid function.)

There are a number of conditions that can affect the thyroid, its function, and its structure.

Hypothyroidism/Underactive Thyroid

Hypothyroidism is a condition of too little thyroid hormone. This lack of hormone can be due to a thyroid that isn't producing enough hormone, a thyroid that has been radioactively treated (which effectively makes it nonfunctional), a thyroid that is affected by drugs and nutritional deficiencies, or a thyroid that is incapable of functioning properly due to nodules, infection, or atrophy. In some cases, the thyroid is surgically removed—all or in part—as a treatment for cancer, nodules, goiter, or hyperthyroidism, leaving most patients permanently hypothyroid. A small number of people have congenital hypothyroidism, meaning they were born without a functional thyroid.

Symptoms of hypothyroidism tend to mirror the slowed metabolism that results from insufficient thyroid hormone. They include fatigue, weight gain, constipation, fuzzy thinking, depression, body pain, and slow reflexes.

Conventional hypothyroidism treatment typically involves replacing the missing thyroid hormone, using prescription thyroid hormone replacement drugs, such as levothyroxine (brand names Synthroid, Levoxyl, Levothroid, and Unithroid), or natural desiccated thyroid drugs, such as Armour and Nature-Throid. Holistic and integrative treatments often focus on nutritional support, supplementation with thyroid precursors like tyrosine and iodine, and adrenal support.

Hyperthyroidism/Overactive Thyroid: Thyrotoxicosis

Thyrotoxicosis refers to the various effects of exposure to too much thyroid hormone. Hyperthyroidism implies that this excess of hormones originated in the thyroid gland itself (and not, for example, from taking an excess of thyroid medication). Hyperthyroidism can be caused by a number of thyroid problems, including autoimmune thyroid disease, nodules that independently produce thyroid hormone, infection, and other causes.

Symptoms of hyperthyroidism tend to mirror the rapid metabolism that results from an oversupply of thyroid hormone. They include anxiety, insomnia, rapid weight loss, diarrhea, high heart rate, high blood pressure, eye sensitivity/bulging, and vision disturbances.

Conventional treatment in the United States focuses on disabling the thyroid permanently, by administering radioactive iodine (RAI) treatment, which renders most patients hypothyroid for life. Some physicians in the United States use prescription antithyroid drugs such as propylthiouracil (PTU) and methimazole (brand name Tapazole) and beta blockers to calm down the thyroid and the immune system, with the hope of remission of the disease, which occurs in as many as 30 percent of patients. Antithyroid drugs are the first choice, however, for doctors outside the United States. In rarer cases, and more commonly outside the United States, surgery to remove the thyroid is used to treat an overactive thyroid. Ultimately, most people with Graves' disease and hyperthyroidism treated conventionally end up hypothyroid for life as a result of RAI or surgery.

Holistic and integrative treatments prior to RAI or surgery focus on supplementing antithyroid drug approaches with natural antithyroid foods, supplements, and herbs that have no side effects, as well as calming and rebalancing the immune system through nutrition, herbs, supplements, movement therapy such as yoga, and energy work.

Goiter/Enlargement

Goiter is the term used to describe an enlargement of the thyroid gland. The thyroid gland can enlarge as a response to insufficient or excessive iodine, thyroid inflammation or infection, or autoimmune disease. The thyroid becomes large enough so that it can be seen on ultrasounds or x-rays and may visibly thicken the neck. Symptoms of goiter include a swollen, tender, or tight feeling in the neck or throat, hoarseness or coughing, and difficulty swallowing or breathing.

Treatment for goiter depends on how enlarged the thyroid has become, as well as other symptoms. It can include observation and monitoring of a smaller goiter that isn't causing symptoms, thyroid hormone replacement medication to help shrink the goiter, aspirin or corticosteroid drugs to shrink thyroid inflammation, and surgery for a goiter that is affecting breathing or swallowing or is cosmetically unattractive.

Nodules/Lumps

Many people have nodules in the thyroid, but you typically can't feel most of them externally. In many cases, nodules aren't functioning and cause no symptoms, and they require only periodic monitoring. Some nodules impair the thyroid's ability to function properly and cause hypothyroidism. Others can become overactive and produce thyroid hormone on their own; these are called "toxic nodules" and can trigger hyperthyroidism. Very large nodules can compromise breathing or swallowing. A very small percentage of nodules are cancerous.

Symptoms of nodules depend on function, size, and location. Nodules that are producing thyroid hormone can trigger hyperthyroidism symptoms, such as palpitations, insomnia, weight loss, anxiety, and tremors. Nodules that are impairing thyroid function can also trigger hypothyroidism symptoms, such as weight gain, fatigue, and depression. Larger nodules that are pressing on the windpipe (trachea), esophagus, or vocal cords can cause difficulty swallowing, difficulty breathing, pain or pressure in the neck, a hoarse voice, or neck tenderness. Some nodules cause no symptoms at all.

Nodules that aren't causing symptoms may be left alone and periodically monitored, or they can be treated with thyroid hormone replacement to help shrink them. Typically, nodules are surgically removed if they are causing difficulties with breathing, swallowing, or speaking or if test results indicate a suspected malignancy.

THYROID DISEASES

A variety of diseases can affect the thyroid and trigger thyroid conditions, such as hypothyroidism, hyperthyroidism, nodules, and goiter.

Hashimoto's Disease and Thyroiditis

There are two different autoimmune diseases in which an immune system dysfunction targets the thyroid: Hashimoto's disease and Graves' disease. In the United States, the vast majority of thyroid conditions are the result of an autoimmune disease.

Hashimoto's disease is the most common form of thyroiditis, an inflammation of the thyroid, so the condition is also often referred to as Hashimoto's thyroiditis. It is the most common thyroid problem and is the cause of most hypothyroidism in the United States. In Hashimoto's, antibodies react against proteins in the thyroid, causing gradual destruction of the gland. Occasionally, before the thyroid is destroyed, it has thyrotoxic periods—known as hashitoxicosis—during which the thyroid overproduces thyroid hormone. Eventually the gland is destroyed and becomes unable to produce thyroid hormones.

Symptoms of Hashimoto's disease can include pain and tenderness in the thyroid area, neck, and throat, difficulty sleeping, and, usually, hypothyroidism. Typically, treatment is for hypothyroidism and involves lifelong thyroid hormone replacement. Holistic and integrative approaches tend to look at healing the underlying autoimmune imbalance and may include nutritional support for the thyroid (selenium, tyrosine, B vitamins, etc.), elimination of toxins and stress, and overall support for the immune system.

Graves' Disease

Graves' disease (sometimes referred to as diffuse toxic goiter because of the typical presence of a goiter) usually causes hyperthyroidism. In the United States, it's thought that Graves' disease and hyperthyroidism affect slightly less than 1 percent of the population, or slightly less than 2.9 million people. Some experts believe, however, that as many as 4 percent of Americans, or 11.8 million people, may have a mild form of Graves' disease, with few symptoms.

In Graves' disease, antibodies bind to the gland, causing the thyroid to overproduce thyroid hormone and resulting in hyperthyroidism. Treatment for Graves' disease follows hyperthyroidism treatment and usually includes antithyroid drugs, radioactive iodine ablation, or surgical removal of the thyroid. Most Graves' disease patients end up hypothyroid over time, requiring lifelong thyroid hormone replacement. Holistic and integrative treatment approaches to Graves' disease often include herbal remedies, nutritional support for the thyroid and immune system, elimination of toxins, and stress reduction approaches.

Thyroid Cancer

Thyroid cancer is one of the least common cancers in the United States but is the most common of endocrine cancers. It is also one of the only cancers whose incidence in the United States has been on the rise in recent years. The American Cancer Society estimates that there are more than 37,000 new cases of thyroid cancer diagnosed each year and more than 1,500 thyroid cancer deaths annually.

Treatment and prognosis depend on the type of thyroid cancer. An estimated 80 to 90 percent of thyroid cancers are papillary or follicular in nature, and most can be treated successfully when discovered early. Medullary thyroid carcinoma makes up 5 to 10 percent of all thyroid cancers and has a good cure rate if discovered before it spreads. Anaplastic thyroid carcinoma is quite rare, accounting for only 1 to 2 percent of all thyroid cancers, and tends to be aggressive and the least likely to respond to treatments.

Although many thyroid cancer sufferers have no symptoms at first, some develop a lump in the neck, voice changes, difficulty breathing or swallowing, or swelling in the lymph nodes.

Treating thyroid cancer almost always involves surgery to remove the thyroid and cancerous lymph nodes. RAI therapy is also given after surgery to kill any remaining cancer cells. Hormone therapy, using thyroid hormone drugs, is frequently used to stop cancer cells from growing.

Because the entire thyroid is removed as treatment for most thyroid cancers, almost all thyroid cancer survivors end up hypothyroid and need to take thyroid replacement hormone for life. Their medication needs to be at a high enough dose to ensure that their TSH levels remain low (nearly undetectable, actually) to help prevent a relapse of cancer. Survivors are regularly checked for reoccurrence.

Risk Factors for Thyroid Conditions

AGE

Thyroid problems become more prevalent as women age. The American Association of Clinical Endocrinologists (AACE Web site) states that thyroid problems affect one in eight women ages thirty-five to sixty-five and one in five women—20 percent—over age sixty-five. Some experts believe that the prevalence is much higher, and recommendations to narrow the TSH range could qualify as many as sixty million Americans, most of them adult women, as having thyroid conditions.

GENETICS/HEREDITY/MEDICAL HISTORY

There is a greater risk of developing a thyroid condition if you have a parent, sibling, or child with any thyroid condition, including autoimmune thyroid problems like Hashimoto's and Graves' disease, nodules, goiters, or thyroid cancer. Up to 50 percent of first-degree relatives of people with autoimmune thyroid disease will themselves have thyroid antibodies that may predispose them to develop autoimmune hypothyroidism. In addition to thyroid issues, a personal or family history of other autoimmune or endocrine diseases also slightly increases your risk of developing autoimmune thyroid disease. In particular, there are higher risks for thyroid conditions among people who have a personal or family history of

- Pituitary tumors
- Celiac disease (intolerance/allergy to gluten and wheat)
- Insulin-dependent (type 1) diabetes
- Addison's disease (a lack of adrenal hormones)
- Cushing's disease (an excess of adrenal hormones)
- Polycystic ovary syndrome (a condition that causes insulin resistance and type 2 diabetes, weight gain, hair loss, and infertility)
- Premature ovarian decline/premature ovarian failure

- **Alopecia** (a condition that causes hair loss, ranging from small patches to total body hair loss)
- **Raynaud's disease** (a condition that causes numbness and tingling in the extremities and sometimes causes fingers or toes to turn blue or white and suffer reduced circulation)
- **Sjögren's syndrome** (a condition that causes severe dry eyes and dry mouth)
- **Rheumatoid arthritis**
- **Systemic lupus erythematosus** (also known as lupus)
- **Multiple sclerosis**
- **Sarcoidosis** (a condition that causes inflammation and lumps in cells and can cause permanent organ damage)
- **Scleroderma** (a condition that causes hardening in the skin or other organs and can cause permanent organ damage)
- **Vitiligo** (a condition that causes loss of pigment in the skin, resulting in irregular, pale patches)
- **Psoriasis**

Left-handedness, ambidextrousness, and prematurely gray hair are considered genetic markers for an increased risk of autoimmune disease, including thyroid problems.

CIGARETTE SMOKING

Women who are current or former smokers have an increased risk of hypothyroidism. Cigarettes contain a chemical, thiocyanate, that adversely affects the thyroid gland and acts as an antithyroid agent, slowing down the thyroid. Smoking can also aggravate some Graves' disease and hyperthyroidism symptoms, especially thyroid eye-related problems.

RECENT PREGNANCY OR MISCARRIAGE

Having had a baby in the past year puts women at an increased risk of developing thyroid problems, including the short-term condition known as postpartum thyroiditis. Some doctors estimate that as many as 10 percent of women develop a thyroid problem after delivery. While some postpartum cases of hypothyroidism are temporary and resolve within six months to a year after delivery, the period after pregnancy is also a common time for permanent thyroid problems to surface.

Pregnancy that ends in miscarriage can also be associated with an increased risk of the onset of thyroid problems.

IODINE DEFICIENCY/EXCESS

Both a deficiency and an excess of iodine are risk factors for thyroid disease. Iodine deficiency can cause an enlarged thyroid (goiter) and hypothyroidism; it is most common in areas that do not add iodine to salt (that is, iodized salt) and in areas with insufficient iodine in the soil known as "goiter belts." Goiter belt areas include the St. Lawrence river valley; the Appalachian mountains; the Great Lakes basin westward through Minnesota, South Dakota, North Dakota, Montana, Wyoming, southern Canada, the Rockies, and into noncoastal Oregon, Washington, and British Columbia; and the Alps, Pyrenees, Himalayas, and Andes.

Mild iodine deficiency in a pregnant woman can cause cognitive and developmental problems in her children that may reduce a child's IQ by as much as fifteen points. Serious iodine deficiency in a pregnant woman can cause stillbirth, miscarriage, and a congenital abnormality known as cretinism. Cretinism is a serious, irreversible condition involving often severe mental retardation and is most common in iodine-deficient areas of Africa and Asia.

Where there is not enough iodine naturally occurring in the food supply, some areas have added iodine to bread or salt to help prevent iodine deficiency. But many people in the world are still iodine-deficient and don't have access to iodization programs. According to the World Health Organization, iodine deficiency is the most prevalent yet easily preventable cause of brain damage. It's common, affecting more than 740 million people, or 13 percent of the world's population. An additional 30 percent of the population is at risk of iodine deficiency-related problems.

About 20 percent of the American public is iodine deficient, but the primary cause of thyroid problems in the United States is auto-immune thyroid disease and is not thought to be iodine-related. In areas like the United States where iodine deficiency is not as common, there is a risk of excessive iodine intake and exposure, from exposure to contrast dye for x-rays or scans, to the use of topical antiseptics like povidone and iodine, to iodine supplements (including bladder wrack, kelp, bugleweed, Irish moss, and seaweed), to the use of the antiarrhythmia drug amiodarone, which contains iodine. In some women, excessive iodine increases the risk of Hashimoto's disease and hypothyroidism. In other women, being exposed to or ingesting an excess of iodine—and, in some cases, simply being exposed to iodine—can trigger hyperthyroidism. This is sometimes referred to as Jod-Basedow, or iodine-induced, thyrotoxicosis.

OVERCONSUMPTION OF GOITROGENIC FOODS

A particular class of foods known as goitrogens can promote thyroid enlargement (goiter) and cause hypothyroidism. These foods have the ability to block the body from using iodine in the production of thyroid hormone. Goitrogens are a concern only for people who still have a thyroid gland that is functional. They are considered most potent when served raw in larger quantities, and studies show that cooking reduces or eliminates much of the goitrogenic potential. A list of some more common goitrogenic foods includes the following:

- Brussels sprouts
- Rutabaga
- Turnips
- Kohlrabi
- Radishes

- Cauliflower
- African cassava
- Millet
- Babassu oil (a palm oil popular in Brazil and Africa)
- Cabbage
- Kale
- Soy products
- Horseradish
- Mustard
- Corn
- Broccoli
- Turnips
- Carrots
- Peaches
- Strawberries
- Peanuts
- Spinach
- Watercress
- Mustard greens
- Walnuts

OVERCONSUMPTION OF SOY PRODUCTS

Soy is also a common goitrogen, but given its popularity as a "health food," in particular, for women in perimenopause/menopause, it deserves its own mention. Soy products have definite antithyroid and goitrogenic effects. There is evidence that long-term overconsumption of soy products can promote formation of goiters and development of autoimmune thyroid disease. Concentrated forms of isoflavone-rich soy (in the form of pills and powders) tend to be more of a risk than fermented food forms, such as tofu, miso, and tempeh.

ENVIRONMENTAL TOXINS

A variety of chemicals in the environment have the ability to affect thyroid function.

Fluoride

Added to drinking water and toothpaste, fluoride is a chemical with strong antithyroid properties that increase the risk of hypothyroidism. In the past, fluoride was used as a drug to treat an overactive thyroid.

Chlorine

Found in chlorinated water supplies and swimming pools, chlorine can interfere with proper thyroid hormone conversion and can increase the risk of hypothyroidism.

Mercury

A component that was used in dental fillings and a toxin found in some fish, mercury can disable the thyroid's ability to convert T4 to T3, resulting in hypothyroidism.

Other heavy metals

Elevated levels of gold, cadmium, and other heavy metals have been linked to an increase in autoimmune thyroid conditions. Heavy metals are sometimes found in water supplies, and some jobs present an exposure risk to these metals.

Perchlorate

This chemical blocks iodine from entering the thyroid and prevents synthesis of thyroid hormone, causing hypothyroidism in some women. Perchlorate is a by-product of rocket and rocket fuel production, and poor disposal, accidents, and use of perchlorate in fertilizers have contaminated water supplies around the United States. Produce grown in those states that use contaminated water for irrigation has reached around the nation.

Dioxins

These chemical compounds are formed through the combination of heat and chlorine and are highly carcinogenic and toxic. They are known to negatively affect thyroid function, and exposure to them increases the risk of hypothyroidism. Dioxins are known to contaminate air and water supplies around the world.

Methyl tertiary butyl ether (MTBE)

This oxygenate is added to gasoline and other chemicals and acts as an "endocrine disrupter."

Insecticides

Several insecticides used to treat airplanes and to eradicate mosquitoes carrying West Nile virus have been shown to have a negative effect on thyroid function. Among these pesticides are resmethrin (brand name Scourge) and sumithrin (brand name Anvil).

X-RAYS, RADIATION, AND RADIUM TREATMENTS

A variety of medical tests and treatments that involve radiation can increase the risk of hypothyroidism. These include:

- X-rays to the head, neck, and chest as a treatment for tonsil, adenoid, lymph node, and thymus gland problems, as well as acne

- Radiation for head, neck, and throat cancers (one study showed that within five years, 48 percent of patients who had received radiation developed hypothyroidism, and within eight years, the projected rate was 67 percent)

- Nasal radium therapy, which involves putting a radioactive rod into the nostril, as a treatment for tonsillitis, colds, and recurrent adenoid problems

NUCLEAR EXPOSURE

Nuclear plants can accidentally release radioactive materials that are damaging to the thyroid. Some nuclear exposure risks:

– Lived in or visited the area near or downwind from the Chernobyl plant in the period after the nuclear accident on April 26, 1986. People at risk included those in Belarus, the Russian Federation, and Ukraine. There was a risk, though reduced, to people in Poland, Austria, Denmark, Finland, Germany, Greece, and Italy.

– Lived near or in the area downwind from the former nuclear weapons plant at Hanford in south-central Washington State during the 1940s through 1960s, particularly 1955 to 1965

– Lived during the 1950s and 1960s in areas subject to fallout from the Nevada Nuclear Test Site northwest of Las Vegas. The fallout was most concentrated in Utah, Idaho, Montana, Colorado, and Missouri. Exposure to this fallout increases the risk of thyroid cancer and autoimmune thyroid disease, particularly in the Farm Belt, where children drank fallout-contaminated milk.

– Lived in the area around the Oak Ridge nuclear facility in eastern Tennessee

INFECTION

Various infections are known to be triggers for some thyroid conditions.

Viral infections, including upper respiratory infections, colds, influenza, mumps, measles, adenovirus, mononucleosis, myocarditis, cat scratch fever, and coxsackie virus, have been implicated as triggers for thyroiditis that can cause hyperthyroidism.

There is also a relationship between *Yersinia enterocolitica* and Hashimoto's thyroiditis. *Yersinia enterocolitica* bacteria are found in the fecal matter of livestock and domesticated and wild animals. You can be exposed to *Yersinia enterocolitica*, therefore, via contaminated meats, especially raw or undercooked products, poultry, unpasteurized milk and dairy products, and seafood (particularly oysters), as well as from sewage-contaminated water and produce fertilized with raw manure. Foods can also be contaminated by food handlers who have not effectively washed their hands before handling food or utensils used to prepare food. Improper storage can contribute to contamination.

SEVERE SNAKEBITE

Not too many people will face life-threatening illness due to snakebite, but it's known that severe snakebite can result in pituitary damage that causes hypothyroidism. This is reported in some people who suffered nearly fatal bites from rare and highly poisonous vipers and rattlesnakes.

MEDICAL/DRUG TREATMENTS

There are certain drugs that are known to cause hypothyroidism in some people who take them. The most common ones are lithium, used to treat bipolar disease and other conditions, and the arrhythmia drug amiodarone (brand name Cordarone). If you are taking these drugs now or have taken them in the past, you are at increased risk for hypothyroidism.

Other drugs that may cause hypothyroidism in some patients are:

- **Glucocorticoids/adrenal steroids** (prednisone and hydrocortisone)
- **Propranolol, a beta blocker**
- **Aminoglutethimide** (used in the treatment of breast and prostate cancer)
- **Ketoconazole, an antifungal**

- **Para-aminosalicylic acid** (used in the treatment of tuberculosis)
- **Sulfonamides** (antibiotics, including sulfadiazine, sulfasoxazole, and acetazolamide)
- **Sulfonylureas, including tolbutamide and chlorpropamide** (used in the treatment of diabetes)
- **Raloxifene** (brand name Evista) (used in the treatment of osteoporosis)
- **Carbamazepine, oxcarbazepine, and valproate** (used in the treatment of epilepsy)

A number of medical treatments and drugs can trigger Graves' disease and/or thyrotoxicosis, including:

- **Interferon beta-1b and interleukin-4**
- **Immunosuppressant therapy**
- **Antiretroviral treatment for AIDS** (acquired immunodeficiency syndrome)
- **Monoclonal antibody** (brand name Campath-1H) **therapy for multiple sclerosis** (a third of patients receiving this treatment develop Graves' disease within six months)
- **Organ donation/bone marrow transplant** (receiving a donated organ or a bone marrow transplant can be a risk for Graves' disease, as the antibodies and lymphocytes can potentially be transferred with the organ or marrow)

Drugs that cause hyperthyroidism as a side effect include the following:

- **Amphetamines**
- **Cimetidine/ranitidine** (brand names Tagamet and Zantac) (used in the treatment of ulcers)
- **Clomiphene** (brand name Clomid) (used in the treatment of infertility)
- **L-dopa inhibitors, such as chlorpromazine** (brand name

Thorazine) and haloperidol (brand name Haldol) (used in the treatment of psychotic disorders)
- Metoclopramide (brand name Reglan) and domperidone (for nausea/vomiting)
- Glucocorticoids/adrenal steroids (prednisone and hydrocortisone)
- Propranolol
- Aminoglutethimide
- Ketoconazole
- Para-aminosalicylic acid
- Sulfonamide drugs, including sulfadiazine, sulfasoxazole, and acetazolamide
- Sulfonylureas, including tolbutamide and chlorpropamide
- Raloxifene (Evista)
- Carbamazepine, oxcarbazepine, and valproate

NECK TRAUMA/WHIPLASH

Research has suggested that trauma to the neck, such as whiplash or a broken neck, can result in hypothyroidism in some people. Researchers speculate that this may be due to injury to and subsequent inflammation of the thyroid tissues themselves. In some patients, trauma to the thyroid or neck area can result in thyrotoxicosis or thyroiditis.

The types of trauma that have been linked to an increased risk of thyroid problems include:

- Recent vigorous manipulation of the thyroid
- Recent vigorous palpation (examination by pressing) of the thyroid
- Recent surgery to the thyroid, parathyroids, or the area surrounding the thyroid
- Recent biopsy of the thyroid
- Recent neck injury (for example, whiplash)
- Recent injection to the thyroid (for example, percutaneous ethanol injection)

ALLERGIES/SENSITIVITIES

A variety of allergies can be risk factors—and possibly triggers—for thyroid problems.

Seasonal allergies to tree pollen can increase antithyroid peroxidase and antithyroglobulin autoantibodies, thus increasing the risk of both Hashimoto's and Graves' disease.

Sensitivity or full intolerance to gluten, found in most wheat and many grain products, is a known trigger of autoimmune disease in general, and in thyroid problems specifically. The condition is known as celiac disease or gluten intolerance.

Some nutritional experts believe that sensitivity or exposure to aspartame (brand name NutraSweet), an artificial sweetener, can contribute to hyperthyroidism.

STRESS

Stress is considered a precipitating factor for some autoimmune diseases. There is evidence that severe emotional or physical stress can trigger the development of Graves' disease. In one analysis, severe emotional stress was seen as the primary precipitating factor in the development of Graves' disease in 14 percent of the patients studied.

RELATED CONDITIONS

Certain conditions are more common in people with Hashimoto's disease and hypothyroidism. While the mechanisms aren't always understood, if you have or have had any of these conditions, you are more likely to develop Hashimoto's disease and become hypothyroid.

- Epstein-Barr virus and mononucleosis
- Carpal tunnel syndrome
- Tarsal tunnel syndrome (an inflammation/irritation/weakness of the shin/lower leg similar to carpal tunnel syndrome)
- Tendinitis
- Plantar fasciitis (a painful inflammatory condition of the foot that causes pain on the underside of the heel)

- Polycystic ovary syndrome
- Mitral valve prolapse (a heart murmur that can cause heart palpitations or skipped beats)
- Down syndrome
- Depression and bipolar disease
- Iron-deficiency anemia
- Hemochromatosis (a condition of excess iron that can cause cirrhosis of the liver, adrenal insufficiency, heart failure, or diabetes)
- Hidradenitis suppurativa (a condition that causes painful, scarring boils in the groin and armpits)
- Urticaria (hives)
- Attention deficit hyperactivity disorder (ADHD)
- Endometriosis
- Candidiasis/yeast overgrowth
- Chronic fatigue syndrome and fibromyalgia
- Type 1 diabetes
- Metabolic syndrome/insulin resistance/type 2 diabetes
- High cholesterol/hyperlipidemia

Certain conditions are more common in people with Graves' disease and hyperthyroidism. Again, how they are connected isn't always clear, but if you have or have had any of these conditions, you are more likely to develop Graves' disease and become hyperthyroid.

- Polyglandular autoimmune syndrome (numerous autoimmune glandular conditions)
- Pituitary gland failure
- Candidiasis/yeast overgrowth
- Malabsorption syndrome (an inability to absorb nutrients from food)
- Chronic active hepatitis
- Type 1 diabetes
- Vitiligo (loss of skin pigmentation)

- Addison's disease
- Pernicious anemia
- Parathyroid gland failure
- Alopecia (hair loss)
- Myasthenia gravis (a condition involving loss of muscle function, especially of the eyes)
- Clinical depression
- Panic disorder/panic attacks
- Phobias
- Generalized anxiety disorder

Thyroid Symptoms

MENSTRUAL IRREGULARITIES

Thyroid problems can cause a variety of menstrual irregularities. Some of the common issues are

- Irregular menstrual cycles and spotting (known as metrorrhagia)
- Shorter cycles, more frequent periods (known as polymenorrhea)
- Longer cycles, less frequent periods (known as oligomenorrhea)
- Heavier, longer, soaking periods (known as menorrhagia)
- No periods at all (known as amenorrhea)
- Lighter periods (known as hypomenorrhea)

INFERTILITY/RECURRENT MISCARRIAGE

Infertility is more common in thyroid patients than in the general population. There are also studies that have shown a linkage between a woman being hypothyroid or hyperthyroid and increased rates of anovulation (failure to release an egg), which contributes to infertility.

Thyroid problems can also increase your risk of miscarriage. Therefore, miscarriage, in particular, recurrent miscarriage, can be considered a "symptom" of thyroid conditions as well.

TEMPERATURE CHANGES: FEELING COLD/HOT

Frequently, an underactive thyroid can cause low body temperature and make you feel cold when it's in fact warm. In particular, hands and feet may feel cold. With hypothyroidism, some women perspire less than normal.

In hyperthyroidism, because of the increase in metabolism, women find themselves feeling warm, or extremely hot, even when it's cold. Some people who are hyperthyroid become intolerant of any warm or hot temperatures and experience hot flashes and excessive sweating.

SLEEP PROBLEMS

Problems with sleep are fairly common in people with an overactive thyroid. Symptoms can include difficulty falling asleep, waking up frequently, and finding it hard to fall back asleep. You may have insomnia and not be able to sleep at all. In both hypothyroidism and hyperthyroidism, some patients are less able to reach deep, restorative stage 4 sleep, so they may wake up feeling tired and unrefreshed. Hypothyroidism also increases the risk of sleep apnea, which can cause frequent waking and can disrupt sleep and cause morning tiredness.

WEIGHT CHANGES

Inappropriate weight gain and the inability to lose weight are very common symptoms of an underactive thyroid. Even mild hypothyroidism, including "normal" TSH levels that are on the higher end of the normal reference range, is associated with weight gain. If you find yourself suddenly gaining weight or unable to lose weight following a reasonable diet (and I don't mean cutting out dessert once a week and expecting to drop pounds and inches!), this may be a symptom of hypothyroidism.

When the body is in a hyperthyroid state, the excess thyroid hormone raises metabolism—enhancing the body's ability to break down fat and muscle—which causes weight loss. Some people don't eat more and haven't changed their exercise habits, yet they lose weight rapidly. Others feel constantly hungry and eat substantially more, yet they either don't gain or lose weight. Some women with hyperthyroidism stop eating or eat very little due to a loss of appetite and are misdiagnosed as being anorexic.

One unique change in hyperthyroidism is an increased appetite for carbohydrates. Researchers have documented that brain chemistry changes in hyperthyroidism actually do increase the appetite, but specifically for carbohydrates far more than for protein and fat.

While the mechanisms aren't well understood, a small percentage of people who are hypothyroid lose weight inappropriately, and a small percentage of people who are actively hyperthyroid gain weight.

MOOD CHANGES

One of the most common symptoms of hypothyroidism is feeling sad or even depressed. You may have feelings of worthlessness, difficulty concentrating, or it may seem as if your mind is "in a fog." You may lose interest in normal daily activities or be more forgetful and have a tougher time keeping up with work, schedules, or details.

Hypothyroidism may also be the reason why your antidepressant doesn't seem to be effective. As many as 80 percent of people on antidepressants may suffer from unresolved symptoms—such as weight gain, lethargy, and loss of libido—that are also very common symptoms of thyroid disease. A significant percentage of people on antidepressants may actually be suffering from undiagnosed thyroid problems.

Some people with hypothyroidism experience increased anxiety. Moods may also change easily, and you might feel restless.

Patients with hyperthyroidism also experience changes to mood and feelings. You may experience swings in mood and emotions, even to the extent that you are behaving erratically or overemotionally. You may have feelings of uncontrollable or irrational anger or feel aggressive for no reason.

Anxiety is even more common in hyperthyroidism, given the elevated heart rate, blood pressure, and racing metabolism. Symptoms can include feeling restless, irritable, on edge, nervous, or inexplicably frightened. You may be worrying all the time and find that you can't stop. You may find yourself jumpy and easily startled and have fast reflexes, tremors, or shaky hands. You may find that you can't sit still and are always moving, jiggling, tapping a foot, or drumming your fingers.

Some people with hyperthyroidism have panic attacks, including the full list of symptoms, such as palpitations, sweating or chills, difficulty breathing, terror, nausea, feeling as if you are going to die, tingling or numbness, dizziness, and faintness. Some patients are incorrectly diagnosed as having panic disorder, when their panic attacks are actually triggered by their hyperthyroid state, and the attacks go away once the thyroid is normalized.

LOSS OF SEX DRIVE

A low sex drive (low libido) is a common symptom of hypothyroidism. Typically, patients with hypothyroidism who have sexual symptoms have low or no desire, problems with arousal, or difficulty having an orgasm. For some people, a sexual problem, in particular, a lack of desire, may be the first noticeable symptom of an underlying thyroid condition.

HAIR LOSS

Hypothyroidism, hyperthyroidism, and autoimmune thyroid disease are all associated with loss of hair—both on the head and on the body. Typically, hair falls out at the root faster than normal and can become brittle, breaking more easily when handled. A unique and noticeable hypothyroidism symptom is loss of the hair from the outer part of the eyebrow.

Your hair can also look and feel very coarse, rough, and dry. In Graves' disease and hyperthyroidism, hair may become thinner, finer, and softer. Women with hypothyroidism and hyperthyroidism often complain that their hair can no longer hold a curl or a perm.

Having autoimmune thyroid problems also puts you at higher risk of developing hair loss due to the autoimmune condition alopecia.

SKIN CHANGES

Changes to the skin associated with hypothyroidism include

- Pale hue
- Dry mucous membranes
- Easy bruising
- Yellowish cast
- Cracked skin on elbows and kneecaps
- Hives or chronic urticaria
- Chronic itching
- Psoriasis
- Eczema
- Hidradinitis suppurativa

Interestingly, because the increased metabolism causes more rapid turnover of skin cells, women with hyperthyroidism may find their skin smoother, younger looking, even velvety.

More often, however, people report a variety of skin problems, including worsening acne; bruising; spider veins on the face and neck; blisterlike bumps on the forehead and face (called "miliaria bumps"); a flushed appearance to the face, throat, palms, and elbows; and sometimes a yellowish cast to their skin.

Hives and itching are frequent symptoms of people with Graves' disease and thyrotoxicosis.

A loss of skin pigmentation, known as vitiligo, can also be a symptom.

One unusual skin condition seen in people with Graves' disease is pretibial myxedema (also known as dermopathy, infiltrative dermopathy, or sometimes Graves' dermopathy). If you develop pretibial myxedema, you may notice waxy, red-brown lesions on your shins and lower legs that are itchy and inflamed. These lesions typically heal into rough, leathery patches. Occasionally, pretibial myxedema can affect the tops of your feet, as well as your toes, arms, face, shoulders, or trunk.

BONE LOSS

Women who had lengthy periods of untreated hyperthyroidism due to Graves' disease are at risk of lower bone mineral density, which increases the risk of osteoporosis.

Some practitioners believe that chronic hypothyroidism, because it slows the metabolism and impairs bone formation, may also be associated with risks of lower bone mineral density.

ELEVATED CHOLESTEROL LEVELS

Elevated cholesterol levels, in particular, elevated cholesterol that does not respond to cholesterol-lowering medication, is a common symptom of hypothyroidism.

Less commonly, hyperthyroidism can cause unusually low cholesterol levels in some women.

FATIGUE, LACK OF ENERGY

However you describe it, fatigue, exhaustion, weakness, lethargy, or feeling run down, sluggish, overtired is one of the most common thyroid symptoms. You may find yourself needing a nap in the afternoon just to make it to dinnertime. You may sleep ten or twelve hours a night and still wake up exhausted. You may find yourself less able to exercise, and your endurance drops because of weakness or lethargy. Or you just walk around feeling exhausted on the same amount of sleep that used to leave you feeling refreshed.

ACHES AND PAINS

Many thyroid patients, both hypothyroid and hyperthyroid, experience chronic pain, aches, and stiffness in various joints and muscles, particularly the hands and feet. The aches and pains can sometimes be so severe that doctors mistake them for arthritis symptoms, and there is a higher incidence of fibromyalgia in thyroid patients.

Carpal tunnel syndrome (which causes pain and weakness in the forearms, hands, and fingers), tarsal tunnel syndrome (which causes pain in the calves, shins, and feet), and plantar fasciitis (which causes pain in the soles of the feet) are all associated with untreated or undertreated hypothyroidism.

In hyperthyroidism, you may feel muscle weakness, especially in the upper arms and legs.

GASTROINTESTINAL/DIGESTIVE DISTURBANCES

Constipation is a common symptom of hypothyroidism. Often, this type of constipation does not respond to increased dietary fiber, increased water consumption, laxatives, and fiber products like Metamucil.

It's common for people with hyperthyroidism to report having more frequent bowel movements, looser bowel movements, or even diarrhea. You may also find that you have to urinate more frequently. A smaller percentage of people experience nausea and/or vomiting as a symptom.

Ascites, an abnormal accumulation of fluid in the abdomen, can be a sign of hypothyroidism. Symptoms of ascites include rapid weight gain, abdominal distention, shortness of breath, and swollen ankles.

Some thyroid patients also report pain in the upper right abdominal area, which may be due to adrenal inflammation or costochondritis, an inflammation of the cartilage that connects rib to breastbone.

DRYNESS

Dry eyes and dry mouth can be symptoms of thyroid disease. Because thyroid disease is frequently autoimmune in nature, thyroid patients have a higher incidence of Sjögren's syndrome, which can cause severe dry mouth and increased cavities, and dry eye symptoms, including pain, light sensitivity, and irritation.

BREAST CHANGES

Some people with hypothyroidism have imbalances in prolactin, the hormone that controls breastfeeding. One symptom that can signal hypothyroidism is lactation, or milk leaking from breasts, in a woman who otherwise is not breastfeeding.

HEART/BLOOD PRESSURE-RELATED SYMPTOMS

Heart and blood pressure changes are often symptomatic of both hypothyroidism and hyperthyroidism.

In hypothyroidism, some women have palpitations (irregular heart rhythms). Some women with hypothyroidism have a slowed heart rate and low blood pressure, but paradoxically, others actually experience high blood pressure when hypothyroid.

In hyperthyroidism, women may experience flutters, noticeable skipped beats, or a strange pattern or heart rate rhythm. You may have a headache and feel breathless, even dizzy. Some people feel a twinge of pain, specifically pain in the chest. Typical symptoms include a feeling that your heart is racing and pounding. If you take your pulse, you may find it over one hundred beats per minute. You may feel as if you can "hear" your heartbeat in your head.

CONCENTRATION AND MEMORY PROBLEMS

Many women with thyroid disease notice changes in thinking as a symptom.

Some of the most commonly reported symptoms are difficulty concentrating, difficulty making decisions, confusion, memory problems, and feeling as if your thinking is disorganized. You may have dyslexia or difficulty with reading, calculating, and thinking. You may have memory problems, find yourself forgetting things more frequently, or feel that your mind is going blank all the time.

You may also feel as if your mind is always racing and you can't shut your thoughts off.

Some people refer to it as "brain fog," that fuzzy feeling that makes it difficult to concentrate.

HEADACHES/MIGRAINES

Worsening of chronic headaches and/or migraine disease can be a symptom of thyroid disease.

INABILITY TO TOLERATE MEDICINES, DRUGS, AND TOXINS

Because hypothyroidism slows down the metabolism and the liver's ability to process toxins, some people find that they are unable to tolerate medicines, alcohol, coffee, and toxins without experiencing side effects. Alexandria, Virginia, physician Donna Hurlock, who works with many thyroid patients, has said that she notices that many of her thyroid patients find that even small doses of medication have greater side effects, even small amounts of caffeine make them jittery, and they feel that alcohol has a stronger effect.

PULSE AND BLOOD PRESSURE CHANGES

Pulse, or heart rate, varies depending on age, level of fitness, and other factors. But, generally, an average heart rate/pulse runs around sixty to eighty-five beats per minute. Athletes and those taking some medications may have a slower heart rate, but a slowed heart rate can also be a symptom of an underactive thyroid. An elevated pulse rate can be a sign of an overactive thyroid.

Similarly, lower blood pressure can be a sign of an underactive thyroid, and high blood pressure can be a sign of hyperthyroidism.

EYE PROBLEMS

The eyes are a frequent target for thyroid symptoms. The majority of problems are in women with Graves' disease and hyperthyroidism, which can cause a variety of eye-related symptoms, including sensitivity, swelling, and blurred vision. Some Graves' patients have an additional, related problem, thyroid eye disease, which is also known as Graves' ophthalmopathy or thyroid-associated ophthalmopathy (TAO). Thyroid eye disease is an inflammation of the eyes and bulging or protrusion of the eyeballs (the medical term is exophthalmos), blurred or diminished vision, red or inflamed eyes, and double vision.

Eye movement can be affected, and one of the characteristic eye changes is called "lid lag." In lid lag, the upper eyelid doesn't follow smoothly along when you look down. The appearance of the eyes also can change, and the eyes may appear red, with visible blood vessels. The upper and lower eyelids may look irritated and puffy, and you may have a noticeable stare. The upper eyelids may retract, giving you a wide-eyed, startled look.

While thyroid eye disease is associated with Graves' disease, both hypothyroidism and hyperthyroidism are associated with a variety of other eye symptoms, including:

- Eyes that feel gritty and dry
- Eyes that are photosensitive (sensitive to light)
- Eyes that have more frequent tics (referred to as nystagmus)
- Headaches due to eye sensitivity
- Eyes that are dry and blurry

NECK AND THROAT COMPLAINTS

Both hypothyroid and hyperthyroid patients can have problems in the neck and throat area, including:

- Thyroid/neck enlargement (goiter)
- A feeling of fullness or pressure in the neck/throat
- Discomfort with neckties, necklaces, turtlenecks, or scarves
- A choking sensation, as if something is stuck in your throat

- Hoarseness
- Difficulty swallowing
- Tongue feels thick

Goiter is one of the most common symptoms in people with Graves' disease. Some women with Graves' disease also report a peculiar, "buzzy" feeling in the neck/thyroid area, as if a low current of electricity is running through it or as if the thyroid is vibrating.

HEARING ISSUES

Tinnitus, commonly referred to as "ringing in the ears," is the perception that you're hearing hissing, roaring, whistling, clicking, ringing, or other noise when there is no sound. Tinnitus can be a symptom of hypothyroidism in some women.

Hearing loss, including sudden onset of hearing loss and deafness, is reported to be related to hypothyroidism in some people, although it's considered a very rare symptom.

BREATHING DIFFICULTIES, ASTHMALIKE FEELINGS, SLEEP APNEA, AND SNORING

Sleep apnea involves momentary lapses of breathing while sleeping and is accompanied by loud snoring, snoring and gasping for breath as you sleep, and feeling tired all the time, no matter how much sleep you get. It can be a symptom of hypothyroidism. In fact, undiagnosed and improperly treated hypothyroidism is considered an important but frequently overlooked cause of sleep apnea.

While not reported in patient literature, a hypothyroidism symptom that many people have reported to me—and one I experienced myself—is a feeling of shortness of breath and tightness in the chest. Some people describe this as "feeling like I need to yawn just to get enough oxygen." Sometimes this can be mistaken for asthma. Some practitioners have speculated that this is due to insufficient oxygen circulation due to hypothyroidism.

NAILS/HANDS

Dry, brittle nails that break easily are more common in people with hypothyroidism.

In hyperthyroidism, nails may be more shiny than usual and break easily because they are softer. The palms may be warm and moist. Two unusual conditions can be seen in some patients with hyperthyroidism. In the first, acropachy, or thyroid acropachy, the fingertips and toes swell and become wider, sometimes even clubbed. This can be accompanied by arthritic damage to the joints in the fingers and/or toes. In the second condition, onycholysis, also called Plummer's nails, the underlying nail bed separates from the skin.

LOW, HUSKY, HOARSE VOICE

Changes in voice are frequently associated with hypothyroidism. Most typically, the voice becomes hoarse, husky, or gravelly. (Some women have even reported that when hypothyroid, they are mistaken for a man on the phone.)

ALLERGIES

Development of allergies or worsening of existing allergies— including hay fever, seasonal allergies, and food allergies—have all been reported as symptoms of hypothyroidism.

DIZZINESS AND VERTIGO

Vertigo is dizziness with the illusion of motion. When you have vertigo, you may feel you are moving or that things are moving around you. Lightheadedness, dizziness, and vertigo can all be symptoms of both hypothyroidism and hyperthyroidism.

PUFFINESS AND SWELLING

Swelling, bloating, water retention, and puffiness (referred to as edema) of various parts of the body are associated with hypothyroidism. In particular, puffiness and swelling may affect the eyes, eyelids, face, feet, and hands.

SLOWNESS

Slowness in movement and speech is considered a symptom of hypothyroidism.

LOW RESISTANCE/FREQUENT INFECTIONS

Some doctors believe that more frequent infections and less resistance to infection—signs of lowered immunity—are symptoms of hypothyroidism. Many people with thyroid problems also report getting colds, flus, and sinus infections more frequently and have a longer, harder time recuperating from these infections.

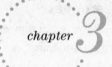
Could It Be
PERIMENOPAUSE OR MENOPAUSE?

It has begun to occur to me that life is a stage I'm going through.

—*Ellen Goodman*

The Menstrual Cycle

To understand perimenopause and menopause, it's essential to understand exactly how your reproductive hormonal cycle works. Many of us think we understand: the egg develops; the uterine lining builds up; the egg is released; if the egg isn't fertilized, you shed the lining; that's your period, and then the whole thing starts again. But it's a much more sophisticated interrelationship of the hormones that keeps the whole cycle moving and in balance.

IN THE BEGINNING

When a girl is born, she has hundreds of thousands of immature eggs in her ovaries. These are all the eggs she will ever have.

From the age of around eight to ten the body starts producing androgens, hormones that trigger the onset of puberty. The beginning of breast development signals the start of puberty, usually followed by the appearance of pubic and underarm hair and breast buds. Around six months before the first menstrual period, vaginal discharge also frequently appears.

The first menstrual period usually occurs around twenty-four to thirty months after puberty starts, but it can start as early as a year and as late as three years. Usually, the first menstrual period won't occur until a girl has reached around one hundred pounds and has approximately 25 percent body fat. This happens, on average, around age twelve or thirteen for most girls.

The process that triggers the first menstrual period begins when the hypothalamus sends out its first burst of gonadotropin-releasing hormone (GnRH). GnRH goes to the pituitary gland, where it triggers the pituitary to release two key hormones: luteinizing hormone (LH) and follicle-stimulating hormone (FSH). FSH and LH in turn go to the ovaries, where they stimulate one ovary to ovulate and begin producing estrogen. Estrogen, FSH, and LH then set into motion the hormonal cycle that causes the ovary to ovulate, to release its first egg. This begins the first menstrual cycle.

THE MONTHLY CYCLE

Each ovary contains follicles—sacs—and each follicle is filled with eggs. On the first day of the menstrual cycle (referred to as day 1), the follicular phase of the cycle begins. During this phase, estrogen and progesterone are at their lowest levels. These low levels are a signal to the pituitary to begin the menstrual cycle by releasing FSH. As FSH rises, it stimulates the follicles and causes the eggs to mature. How many actual follicles develop each month is not a fixed number and is unique to each woman.

By days 5 to 7, one of these follicles responds to FSH stimulation more than the others and becomes dominant, growing faster than the other follicles. (Occasionally, with higher FSH levels, additional folli-cles may become dominant; this is what can cause multiple births.)

As the egg ripens inside the follicle, the follicle itself secretes estrogen, which stimulates the uterine lining to thicken and get ready for a fertilized egg). Around day 13 of the cycle, the estrogen level reaches a point where it triggers a rapid release (known as a surge) of LH. The body temperature rises for a short time. The surge of LH sets into motion the final maturation of the egg and causes the dominant follicle to force its way to the surface of the ovary to re-lease the egg. (The LH surge is what is measured by home ovulation detection kits.)

Around day 14, the follicle ruptures, and an egg bursts out into the fallopian tube heading to the uterus, a process known as ovula-tion. Typically, ovulation occurs between twenty-eight and thirty-six hours after the LH surge and about twelve hours after LH reaches peak levels.

Around ovulation, the rise in estrogen makes cervical fluid stringy and sticky and more hospitable to sperm, therefore more conducive for conception. The cervix itself becomes softer and more open, again, making conception more possible.

After the egg is released, it's swept into the fallopian tube, and if it is fertilized, this usually takes place while the egg is still in the fallopian tube.

In the meantime, as estrogen levels have been increasing, FSH production is suppressed, and FSH levels decrease.

The nondominant follicles wither away and are reabsorbed. After the dominant follicle ruptures, it collapses and becomes the corpus luteum. The corpus luteum then secretes large amounts of progesterone and some estrogen, which help prepare the uterine lining for implantation of the fertilized egg (an embryo). This built-up uterine lining is known as the endometrium.

The point of ovulation signals the end of the follicular phase and the start of the luteal phase of the menstrual cycle. During this second half of the cycle, which normally runs anywhere from twelve to fifteen days, the body is attempting to support a pregnancy if one occurs.

If the egg is fertilized, a small amount of the hormone called human chorionic gonadotropin (HCG) is released. (HCG, which can be detected as early as seven days after fertilization, is what is measured using early pregnancy tests.) HCG also keeps the corpus luteum viable, so it can continue to produce estrogen and progesterone to maintain the uterine lining.

If the egg was fertilized, it begins to divide and continues toward the uterus, where it may implant itself in the uterine lining. It then continues to grow into a fetus and, ultimately, a baby.

If, as in most cycles, pregnancy does not occur, around ten days after ovulation, the corpus luteum starts to disintegrate, and estrogen and progesterone levels drop.

As estrogen and progesterone levels fall sharply, days 26 to 28 can be referred to as the premenstrual phase. This is when premenstrual syndrome (PMS) is most common.

When the follicle has self-destructed completely, the drop in progesterone triggers the shedding of the endometrium as menstrual bleeding, typically starting on day 28—about 14 days after ovulation.

The time when you are bleeding, or the menstrual phase, can last from one to eight days, but the average is four or five days. The length of the bleeding period tends to remain about the same in women from month to month, but over time, it may change, becoming longer or shorter. The amount of blood lost in each menstruation tends to be similar from cycle to cycle in many women, but it can change over time and become heavier or lighter.

On the first day of menstrual bleeding—often the twenty-eighth day of the cycle—the low estrogen and progesterone levels trigger the pituitary to release FSH and start the cycle again. Day 1 of the new cycle begins.

When the entire system is working properly, the follicular phase (maturation of the egg) takes about fourteen days, and the corpus luteum, which defines the luteal phase, has a life span of approximately fourteen days. This gives the typical woman a menstrual cycle of twenty-eight days, with ovulation typically occurring around the midpoint on day 14.

- **Cycle day 1**
  - menstrual period begins

- **Cycle days 1 to 14**
  - follicular phase

- **Cycle day 14**
  - ovulation

- **Cycle days 14 to 18**
  - luteal phase

- **Cycle days 26 to 28**
  - premenstrual phase

- **Cycle day 28/cycle day 1**
  - menstrual period begins

Each woman's cycle is unique and may not fit this "typical" twenty-eight-day schedule. Cycles can range from as little as twenty-one days to forty or more days. For most women, however, the luteal phase runs from around twelve to sixteen days. If a woman has a particularly long cycle, the additional time will usually extend the length of the follicular phase.

The following graphic depicts the regular menstrual cycle.

THE MENSTRUAL CYCLE

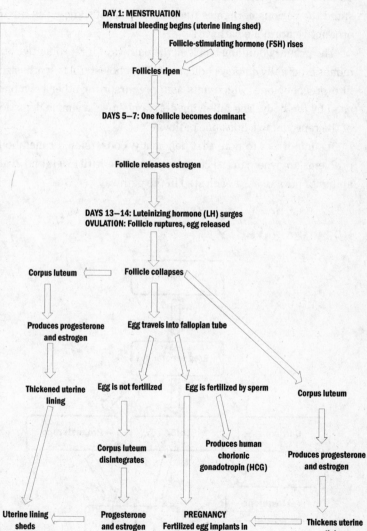

DAY 1: MENSTRUATION
Menstrual bleeding begins (uterine lining shed)

Follicle-stimulating hormone (FSH) rises

Follicles ripen

DAYS 5–7: One follicle becomes dominant

Follicle releases estrogen

DAYS 13–14: Luteinizing hormone (LH) surges
OVULATION: Follicle ruptures, egg released

Follicle collapses

Corpus luteum

Produces progesterone and estrogen

Egg travels into fallopian tube

Thickened uterine lining

Egg is not fertilized

Egg is fertilized by sperm

Corpus luteum

Corpus luteum disintegrates

Produces human chorionic gonadotropin (HCG)

Produces progesterone and estrogen

Uterine lining sheds

Progesterone and estrogen levels drop

PREGNANCY
Fertilized egg implants in thickened uterine lining

Thickens uterine lining

The Reproductive Hormone Pathway

To understand perimenopause/menopause, it's important to understand the various hormones that make up what's known as the reproductive hormone pathway.

The primary building block on the pathway for reproductive hormones is actually dietary cholesterol. The cholesterol is synthesized into pregnenolone, which acts as a precursor for other hormones used by the body. The following diagram shows a simple depiction of the reproductive hormone pathway.

It's important to note that deficiency, conversion, or metabolic problems anywhere in the chain can interfere with levels and availability of hormones at each step in the pathway.

HORMONE PATHWAY

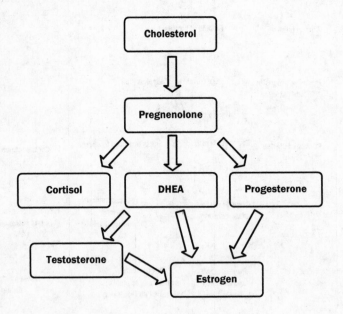

PREGNENOLONE

Pregnenolone is the precursor hormone, synthesized from cholesterol. Pregnenolone is a precursor for three hormones: the adrenal hormone cortisol and the reproductive hormones dehydroepiandrosterone (DHEA) and progesterone. Because it is the precursor for all the other reproductive hormones, pregnenolone is sometimes called the "parent hormone." Pregnenolone has roles in helping to elevate mood and energy, relieve joint pain, and improve concentration and is thought to help with brain function.

DEHYDROEPIANDROSTERONE (DHEA)

DHEA is a steroid hormone produced by the adrenal glands, as well as by the brain and the skin. DHEA levels peak around age twenty-five to thirty and steadily decline after that, so that by age eighty, the DHEA level is typically only about 15 percent of the peak level. DHEA is derived from pregnenolone and broken down into estrogen and testosterone. It helps with memory, the immune system, and muscle strength.

PROGESTERONE

Progesterone is the hormone produced by the corpus luteum of the egg follicle ovaries; after menopause, a small amount is made by the adrenal glands. It is a precursor for estrogen.

The key function of progesterone is to help prepare the uterine lining for a fertilized egg. Progesterone can help enhance mood, promote feelings of calm, and reduce anxiety.

TESTOSTERONE

Testosterone is a male hormone (androgen), but women also produce it in far smaller amounts. It is a precursor for estrogen. For women, testosterone is thought to play a role in libido, arousal, orgasmic response, energy, and muscle building.

ESTROGEN TYPES

There are actually three key types of estrogen in the body: estradiol (known as E2), estrone (E1), and estriol (E3). Estradiol is the main type of estrogen during the reproductive years and is produced by the ovaries. Estriol is the weakest of the estrogens and is made during pregnancy. Estrone is made after menopause and is most commonly found in increased amounts in postmenopausal women. Estrone does the same work in the body that estradiol does, but it is considered weaker in terms of effects.

What Happens in Perimenopause/Menopause

When we're born, our ovaries contain follicles with as many as a million eggs. By puberty, we have around 75,000 to 300,000 eggs remaining. During our reproductive years, about 400 to 500 eggs mature and are released. The rest deteriorate over time.

Perimenopause can naturally start as early as a woman's thirties, but it typically starts in the late thirties/early forties, as progesterone and estrogen levels start to fluctuate.

Perimenopause is triggered when baseline levels of estrogen and progesterone start to decline. At the same time, the supply of egg follicles drops, the follicles that remain are less sensitive to stimulation, and the eggs that remain are old.

Because there are fewer follicles, and because they are less sensitive, the hypothalamus stimulates the pituitary to make more FSH and LH in an attempt to stimulate the remaining follicles, cause them to mature, and trigger an LH surge. FSH levels rise in response.

In some cycles, the follicle doesn't develop fully. Less estrogen is released in those cycles. When estrogen is especially low, it won't trigger an LH surge, and the egg is not released at all. This is known as an anovulatory cycle. In an anovulatory cycle, the follicle doesn't rupture and the corpus luteum isn't produced, so there's no release of progesterone. The drop of estrogen and progesterone levels signals the uterus to shed its lining early, so cycle length shortens and the period comes earlier than usual. (Shorter menstrual cycles and an inability to become pregnant are the most common symptoms of perimenopause.)

In other cycles, the follicle will develop normally, and normal amounts of estrogen and progesterone are released.

As the baseline levels of estrogen and progesterone decline, the monthly changes in these hormones become erratic, and the egg supply dwindles. This causes even more cycles to become anovulatory (no ovulation), and periods come more frequently, usually due to a shortened follicular phase. (The luteal phase tends to remain the same length.)

Cycles when follicles don't develop and progesterone doesn't rise often result in a reduction in PMS symptoms. At the same time, drops in estrogen can cause new symptoms, such as hot flashes and night sweats. As hormone levels drop further, bleeding tends to become heavier and longer and is brown rather than red. Periods can become more erratic, and with more anovulatory cycles, some periods will now be skipped entirely.

As menopause approaches, levels of circulating FSH rise dramatically, in an effort to stimulate the remaining follicles to ovulate. At the same time, the ovaries cut back on production of estrogen.

Eventually, the stock of viable eggs is depleted, and hormone levels cannot trigger ovulation. Menstruation stops, and menopause occurs.

When periods stop entirely—and this can occur hormonally or due to surgical removal of ovaries—there is a fairly dramatic drop in estrogen levels. At this point, the adrenal glands kick in to produce some estrogen. Without a corpus luteum each month, progesterone levels also drop significantly. This is a time when some women, even though estrogen has dropped, develop an imbalance, where the ratio of estrogen to progesterone is high, a condition known as estrogen dominance.

Interestingly, gynecologist and hormone expert Dr. Jerilynn Prior believes that many of the symptoms of perimenopause are actually due to estrogen dominance, not estrogen deficiency, and show signs of high estrogen or insufficient progesterone, including:

- Swollen and tender (sometimes lumpy) breasts
- Increased vaginal mucus and a heavy pelvic feeling, like cramps or swelling
- Heavy flow
- Bleeding at intervals shorter than three weeks
- Continual spotting or flow every two weeks
- Clotting with cramping

Physically, the shifts in estrogen and progesterone can cause a number of observable clinical signs in menopause, including thinning of the vaginal lining, which can make the vagina feel dry or irritated. The bladder lining also thins, which can contribute to more frequent urination, more urinary tract infections, or even incontinence. Fluctuating hormones can also disturb sleep. Skin can lose elasticity, and bone mineral density is frequently reduced.

As far as timing, in the United States, the average age when women have not had a period for a year—menopause—is fifty-one, with the common age range for natural menopause spanning from age forty-eight to fifty-five. Menopause is considered late if it occurs in a woman older than age fifty-five and premature if it occurs before forty.

The clinical "test" for menopause is elevated FSH. But because hormones can fluctuate dramatically, an elevated FSH level in a perimenopausal woman is not enough to confirm menopause. (And importantly, despite FSH levels, a woman can still get pregnant.) Measuring FSH levels can help assess the "progress" toward menopause, but until FSH is consistently elevated to 30 million International Units per milliliter (mIU/mL) or higher and a woman is no longer menstruating, menopause can't be confirmed.

The following flowchart maps out what happens in perimenopause, in particular, why cycles can become shorter.

PERIMENOPAUSAL CYCLE

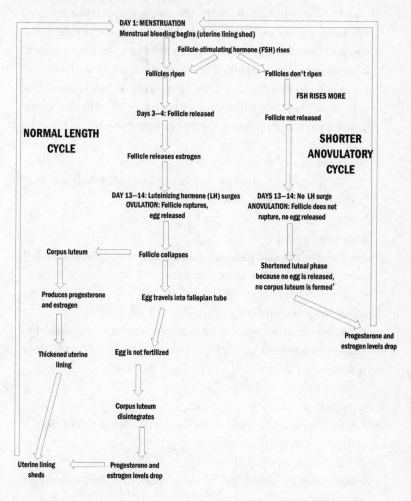

DAY 1: MENSTRUATION
Menstrual bleeding begins (uterine lining shed)

Follicle-stimulating hormone (FSH) rises

Follicles ripen

Follicles don't ripen

FSH RISES MORE

Days 3–4: Follicle released

Follicle not released

NORMAL LENGTH CYCLE

SHORTER ANOVULATORY CYCLE

Follicle releases estrogen

DAY 13–14: Luteinizing hormone (LH) surges
OVULATION: Follicle ruptures,
egg released

DAYS 13–14: No LH surge
ANOVULATION: Follicle does not
rupture, no egg released

Corpus luteum

Follicle collapses

Produces progesterone
and estrogen

Egg travels into fallopian tube

Shortened luteal phase
because no egg is released,
no corpus luteum is formed'

Thickened uterine
lining

Egg is not fertilized

Progesterone and
estrogen levels drop

Corpus luteum
disintegrates

Uterine lining
sheds

Progesterone and
estrogen levels drop

Risk Factors for Menopause

There are a number of factors that are considered "risks" for menopause.

Age

Age is the most obvious risk factor, as the closer a woman is to fifty-one (the most common age for natural menopause), the more at "risk" she is of reaching menopause. As noted before, the common age range for natural menopause spans from age forty-eight to fifty-five, but there are reports of women menstruating into their late fifties and early sixties, as well as women going through natural menopause before age forty.

Genetics/heredity

If your mother or sister had an early or late natural menopause, you are more likely to as well.

Cigarette smoking

Smoking is linked to perimenopause and menopause onset a full two years earlier than in nonsmokers.

Never being pregnant

Never having been pregnant can trigger earlier menopause, because more menstrual cycles deplete the reserve of eggs more quickly.

High altitude

Living at a high altitude is associated with earlier menopause.

Low body weight

Being excessively thin and having a low body weight can trigger an earlier menopause.

Autoimmune disease history

Having a history of autoimmune disease increases your risk of having autoimmune disease of the ovaries (that is, premature ovarian decline or premature ovarian failure), which is associated with early menopause.

Surgery

While removal of both ovaries (bilateral oophorectomy) causes immediate menopause, if the uterus is taken out and one ovary is left, a woman won't have periods, but she may not go through menopause, though she's at a higher risk. Ovarian surgery for adhesions or pelvic endometriosis is also associated with earlier menopause.

Childhood cancer treatment

Receiving chemotherapy or pelvic radiation cancer therapy as a child has been linked to early menopause.

Chemotherapy and radiation therapy

Having chemotherapy and/or radiation therapy to the pelvic region can cause signs and symptoms of menopause, such as hot flashes and cessation of periods, during the course of treatment. In some women, the ovarian function will start after treatment is completed. But in some cases, however, irreparable damage is done to the ovaries, and menopause is triggered.

Radioactive iodine (RAI) treatment for thyroid cancer

Women who have been treated with RAI for thyroid cancer may also experience earlier menopause. In 2001 Italian researchers reported that they'd found that RAI treatment for thyroid cancer provided sufficient radiation to damage ovarian function and follicles, reducing some women's period of fertility and triggering earlier menopause. The patients studied were all younger than age 45 when they received their first treatment for thyroid cancer. The researchers concluded that the RAI treatment was probably a cause of earlier ovarian failure in some thyroid cancer patients.

Polycystic ovary syndrome

This endocrine disorder is associated with earlier menopause.

Extreme athleticism/overexercise

In some women, extreme athleticism or excessive exercise, such as seen in an elite athlete or a marathon runner, is associated with earlier menopause.

Eating disorders/chronic dieting

Eating disorders, such as anorexia and bulimia, and chronic dieting are associated with earlier menopause.

Vegetarianism

Being a vegetarian is associated with earlier menopause.

Drug use

Use of illegal drugs is associated with earlier menopause.

Springtime birth month

It sounds a bit wacky, but there's actually a reputable study that found that women born in March have the earliest menopause, and that women born in October typically reach menopause as much as fifteen months later than women born in the spring. Experts don't know what mechanism is at work; it may be diet during pregnancy, temperature, or seasonal exposure to infections.

Perimenopause/Menopause Terminology

Before we launch into a discussion of what's happening in perimenopause and menopause, let's get the terminology straight, because it can be confusing.

- It's generally agreed by medical experts that *menopause* refers to the point at which you have not had a menstrual period for a full year.

- Depending on who you ask, the time before menopause can be referred to as *perimenopause* or *premenopause*. By some definitions, the perimenopause begins as long as ten years before menopause; others consider it to be the period right before menopause. This period is also sometimes referred to as *menopausal transition* or the *climacteric.* (For decades, women have referred to menopause euphemistically as "the change" or "the change of life.") Many experts agree that the point when hormones start fluctuating erratically actually marks the start of perimenopause, and during perimenopause, menstruation typically continues, although it may not be on a regular cycle.

- **Premature perimenopause:** erratic menstruation and symptoms that occur before age forty are also referred to as premature ovarian decline (POD)
- **Natural menopause:** refers to menopause that happens for natural reasons, that is, loss of ovarian follicular function
- **Surgical menopause:** menopause brought on by surgical removal of both ovaries (bilateral oophorectomy) or, in some cases, removal of one ovary
- **Induced menopause:** menopause brought on by ablation (loss) of ovarian function by chemotherapy or radiation treatments
- **Postmenopause:** the period after the final menstrual period, whether menopause is natural or induced
- **Premature menopause:** natural or induced menopause that occurs before age forty. If natural menopause occurs before age forty, it is referred to as premature ovarian failure.
- **Early menopause:** natural or induced menopause before age fifty-one

Premenopausal/Menopausal Symptoms

There are a number of symptoms commonly associated with perimenopause or menopause. Some are familiar, and others might surprise you.

MENSTRUAL IRREGULARITIES

The most common menopausal symptom, more common even than hot flashes, is an irregular menstrual cycle. Changes in your period are also likely to be one of the first signs that perimenopause is under way.

You may notice changes to typical PMS symptoms. Some women have fewer symptoms during perimenopause. A smaller percentage have worsening PMS during perimenopause.

Earlier in perimenopause, when you are having anovulatory cycles, it's more common to have periods that come more frequently—even every twenty-one days or so.

Later in perimenopause, it's more common to have a longer interval between periods, with many women going thirty-six days or more between periods. In some cases, you may skip a period entirely and pick back up the next month. Some women find that their period stops for a few months, then starts again. Midcycle spotting is also common.

Carolina, like the other women in her family, started her perimenopause in her late thirties.

Now, my periods are becoming longer and longer apart. I went seven months without a period, and then it showed up again this past December. Now I haven't had a period since then, but I don't know if it is because I'm through menopause or if it is going to show up again. It's so hard because you really don't know what is going on or what is causing what.

Some women have what are known as phantom periods. In a phantom period, you have all the signs and symptoms that your period is coming, but it never does.

The length of periods can change as well. If you typically menstruated for five days, you may find that your period gets shorter or longer. Periods can also become lighter or heavier. In fact, a sign that you are getting closer to menopause is that your period may become heavier and last longer. But other women find that they have less menstrual discomfort during perimenopausal periods.

The way the menstrual blood looks also can change. In perimenopause, menstrual blood may take on a brown tinge, and it's not uncommon for the blood to contain heavy clots.

Keep in mind, however, that you can still become pregnant during this period, as you may ovulate during some cycles, and your fertile period may be difficult to predict or identify.

At age forty-six, Anita, who had her thyroid removed, was struggling. Says Anita:

My periods started getting heavy for the first three days. This went on for a while. Then my period started getting really heavy with clots, almost gushing as if I were having a miscarriage to the point where I changed my clothes three or four times a day while wearing two extra long pads. My OB-GYN said nothing was wrong, and it was probably perimenopause. This went on for a while. Then I stopped for about three, almost four months. They did blood work: I was not menopausal. They gave me pills to jump-start my period again. From that point, I was having a period one month, then off two months.

While some bleeding irregularities can be expected during perimenopause, any significant irregular bleeding does need to be evaluated. Some of the causes of abnormal bleeding during perimenopause are

- **Hypothyroidism:** untreated or improperly treated
  hypothyroidism can cause excessive bleeding in some women.
- **Pregnancy:** a normal pregnancy, ectopic pregnancy,
  or miscarriage
- **Fibroids:** noncancerous growths in and around the uterus,
  known as fibroids, can cause bleeding.
- **Uterine lining abnormalities:** polyps in the endometrium

(uterine lining) or overgrowth of the endometrium can cause abnormal bleeding.

- **Cancer**: uterine, vaginal, or cervical cancer is a rare cause of abnormal bleeding.

All postmenopausal bleeding must be evaluated promptly by a physician.

DECREASING FERTILITY/INFERTILITY

Clearly, one of the key symptoms of perimenopause is decreasing fertility. As ovulation becomes less regular, the ability to conceive drops, and after age forty, fertility is estimated to drop by at least 50 percent in most women. The risk of miscarriage after forty is two to three times that of younger women.

As long as you are still having periods—as erratic as they may be—and until you've hit point where it's been at least twelve months since your last period, it is still possible for you to become pregnant. (We've all known someone who had a "change of life" baby.) Women who don't want to become pregnant still need to use birth control during this time.

HOT FLASHES/NIGHT SWEATS

Cartoonist and writer Dee Adams runs the wonderful Minnie Pauz Web site, which features a selection of hilarious cartoons about menopause. What topic has the most cartoons dedicated to it? Hot flashes, of course!

Hot flashes (also known as hot flushes) and their evening counterpart, night sweats, are perhaps the most iconic symptoms of menopause. Together, hot flashes and night sweats are referred to as the climacteric syndrome and vasomotor symptoms.

It's estimated that 75 to 85 percent of women experience hot flashes and night sweats. After menstrual irregularities, they are the most common perimenopausal symptoms. There appears to be a greater risk of hot flashes in women who have a higher body mass or who are obese, in women who smoke, and in women who don't exercise. Women who suffer from high anxiety report four times the rate of hot flashes compared with those with low anxiety.

Hot flashes tend to occur sporadically and can start several years before any other signs of menopause. They also tend to get worse the further into perimenopause and the closer you are to actual menopause—the last period—and are still common into the first three years after menopause. Generally, however, about 80 percent of women with hot flashes have them for less than two years, and a very small percentage have them for more than five years.

More than 80 percent of women who have hot flashes have them for more than a year, but they gradually decline in frequency and intensity over time. Untreated, most hot flashes do stop spontaneously, although it's estimated that approximately 10 percent of women continue to have hot flashes beyond menopause and even into their seventies.

Hot flashes can range in frequency from hourly, to all day and night, to several a day, to just the occasional flash. The U.S. Food and Drug Administration actually defines "mild" hot flashes as those that occur fewer than seven times a day, on average.

In the United States, hot flashes are more common in African-American and Latina women and less common in Chinese-American and Japanese-American women, versus Causasian women.

Hot flashes are more common in the evening and during hot weather. Some women find that there are certain triggers associated with hot flashes, including caffeine, alcohol (especially red wine), hot drinks, spicy foods, chocolate, refined sugar, and stressful or frightening events.

Some hot flashes start with nausea or a headache, but the typical hot flash begins as a feeling of warmth or heat that starts in the abdomen or bellybutton area and moves up toward the head and face. The rapid sensation of heat then affects the face and upper chest area for anywhere from thirty seconds to five minutes. During the hot flash, skin temperature can go up by as much as ten degrees, and a woman may have sweating of the head and upper body. The face may flush or turn red, and some women get blotchy red patches on the chest, back, and arms. During the hot flash, the heart rate typically goes up as much as seven to fifteen beats per minute, and heart palpitations are common. Some women also have dizziness, light-headedness, and vertigo during a hot flash. After the hot flash is done, the skin temperature returns to normal, which can cause cold chills, heavy sweating, and even shivering in some women.

Hot flashes that occur at night—night sweats—are the main cause of sleep problems and insomnia in perimenopausal and menopausal women. Strong night sweats, which are more likely during the first four hours of sleep, can actually wake a woman out of a deep sleep. Mood symptoms and memory problems are more common in women who have nighttime hot flashes, but experts are not clear on how they are linked. Treating the hot flashes reportedly can help improve memory function in women with hot flashes.

The conventional wisdom is that hot flashes are due to declining estrogen levels. The hypothalamus mistakes low estrogen levels in the body as a drop in body temperature. The message goes out for the blood vessels to rapidly expand. Blood flow to the extremities and skin drops, and skin temperature rises in response.

Gynecologist Jerilynn Prior, MD, who is founder of the Centre for Menstrual Cycle and Ovulation Research in Vancouver, has a theory that it's a bit more complicated than simply "declining estrogen." At her Web site, Dr. Prior writes:

Hot flushes occur in both perimenopause and menopause, yet hormone levels are very different. Why? Hot flushes appear to be caused by dropping estrogen levels when the brain has been exposed to, and gotten "used to," higher estrogen levels. Therefore, the hot flushes in perimenopause occur because of the big swings in estrogen from super-high to merely high, or even from high to normal. In menopause, hot flushes occur because estrogen levels have become low after the normal levels of the menstruating years and the higher levels of perimenopause. Although no one has tracked the life experience of hot flushes within a woman, as opposed to in categories of women, I suspect that most women who are going to get hot flushes—except those with surgical menopause or who stop estrogen therapy—start having them before they are officially menopausal.

Some studies have also found that higher FSH levels are correlated to incidence of hot flashes.

SLEEP PROBLEMS

As discussed earlier, some women who have night sweats have significant sleep problems as a result.

Night sweats can cause frequent waking and insomnia. If women find it difficult to fall back to sleep after waking, they may also suffer from exhaustion, memory problems, and depression as a result.

Decreasing estradiol levels (estradiol is the key form of estrogen) also are associated with trouble falling asleep and frequent waking. Elevated FSH is linked to frequent waking.

Some women have erratic sleep or sleep problems without any night sweats. Some of the common problems are

- Difficulty falling asleep
- Frequent waking
- Waking frequently to urinate
- Inability to go back to sleep after waking
- Waking early

Waking earlier than planned tends to become more common through late perimenopause, but sleep habits improve when women are postmenopausal.

WEIGHT GAIN AND REDISTRIBUTION

During perimenopause and into menopause, many women experience weight gain, a redistribution of body fat, and a decrease in muscle mass. Women find that they may gain weight or that fat is redistributed to the abdomen, waist, hips, and thighs. Other women find that it becomes harder to lose weight or easier to gain.

According to the North American Menopause Society, over the average six years of menopause transition, women typically gain seven pounds and two to three inches at the waist. Another study found that women gain an average of five pounds in the three years before menopause.

There is a biological reason for this weight gain, in that extra fat can help to produce estrogen to replace the estrogen lost during perimenopause.

Researchers believe that specialized estrogen receptors in the hypothalamus may be acting as a master switch that controls food intake, energy expenditure, and body fat distribution. They theorize that dropping estrogen levels may cause women to eat more, burn less energy, gain weight, and redistribute body fat directly to the waist, hips, thighs, and abdomen. It's also theorized that estrogen helps the brain remain sensitive to leptin, a hormone that helps regulate energy intake, energy expenditure, appetite, and metabolism.

Some women in perimenopause and menopause report increased cravings for starchy carbohydrates (bread, potatoes, rice, and pasta) and chocolate, which may also contribute to weight gain. Cravings in menopause haven't been studied extensively, but it's thought that dropping serotonin levels in the brain many intensify cravings for sugary, high-carbohydrate foods. Some menopausal women also report craving caffeine, which may be a result of fatigue or sleep disturbances.

There is some evidence that blood sugar imbalances are more common during perimenopause and menopause.

MOOD CHANGES

Perimenopause/menopause is a time when many women experience a variety of mood changes. Estrogen helps elevate mood, and progesterone is a relaxant. It's thought that imbalances and drops in both hormones affect mood.

Some of the complaints reported by perimenopausal and menopausal women are feeling extreme irritability, tension, anger, rapid mood swings, inability to cope with stress, extreme emotionality (for example, bursting into tears), and anxiety.

The greatest incidence of depression in perimenopausal/menopausal women appears to be in the two years after the last menstruation, but this typically lifts. (Interestingly, research has shown that women tend to be more depressed in their twenties and thirties than during or after menopause.) Surgical menopause is an exception, however, and women have double the rate of depression after surgical menopause, when compared with women experiencing natural menopause.

Women who are experiencing sleep problems, hot flashes, or night sweats are more likely to report mood-related symptoms.

Gynecologist and menopause expert Jan Shifren, MD, says that women should be aware that short bursts of anxiety can be a perimenopausal symptom. Says Dr. Shifren:

> I had a perimenopausal patient who reported that she was not having any hot flashes, and had no history of anxiety or depression. She was having these unusual episodes, however, each lasting around five minutes, where her heart would race and she felt incredibly anxious, and then it would pass. They sounded just like classic hot flashes, except without the heat. I suspected that she was having vasomotor symptoms due to estrogen fluctuating, and it appears to be the case, because after treating her with low-dose estrogen, these episodes disappeared.

VAGINAL/OVARIAN/UTERINE PROBLEMS
When estrogen levels drop, the tissues that line the vagina and vulva become drier, thinner, and less elastic. This causes a variety of symptoms.

From 40 to 60 percent of menopausal women find that they need more time and sexual stimulation in order to become lubricated. It is this reduced lubrication that is responsible for painful intercourse, a condition known as dyspareunia, which is more common in women after menopause.

The dryness and lack of lubrication can also result in itching and burning. Women also become more susceptible to vaginal infections. The pH of the vagina changes, shifting from acidic to alkaline, which makes it more susceptible to infections, including atrophic vaginitis and bacterial vaginosis (which can cause a fishy odor and discharge).

Because of the thinness of the vaginal tissue, some women have light spotting after sex.

About 30 percent of women report these sorts of vaginal symptoms during the early postmenopausal period, and almost half complain of these problems after menopause. Unlike hot flashes, vaginal symptoms generally persist, and they tend to get worse with aging.

There is also an increased incidence of ovarian problems, including benign ovarian cysts and fibroids, during perimenopause and menopause.

Women can lose some tone in the pelvis, and this can result in a drop (known as a prolapse) in the reproductive and urinary tract organs, such as the uterus and bladder. Prolapse can cause a feeling of pressure in the vagina, as well as pain and pressure in the lower back.

BLADDER/URINARY PROBLEMS

During perimenopause and after menopause, as estrogen drops, the tissues in the urinary tract and the opening to the bladder (the urethra) also typically become drier, thinner, weaker, and less elastic. This can trigger two key symptoms: incontinence and infection.

Incontinence refers to the involuntary loss or leaking of urine. Among women in menopause, it's estimated that as many as half of all women have some mild problem with incontinence, and 5 to 15 percent have more severe problems.

There are two types of incontinence. "Stress" incontinence refers to leaking urine when coughing, laughing, sneezing, running, or during physical activity. "Urge" incontinence is an intense, sudden urge to urinate that occurs even after emptying the bladder, or a feeling that you have to go to the bathroom all the time. In some cases, a woman may also feel that she can't get to the bathroom quickly enough and begins to leak urine.

In the four or five years after menopause, the thinning of the bladder and urethra causes women to have an increased risk of infections in the urinary tract, including urinary tract infections (UTIs, also known as bladder infections) and cystitis. Symptoms of infection include frequent urination, urinary urgency, difficulty urinating, and a burning sensation when urinating. These infections are treatable with antibiotics, but they tend to recur.

LOSS OF SEX DRIVE

During perimenopause and menopause, the drops in estrogen, progesterone, and testosterone levels can dampen sexual desire, a condition known as loss of libido. In addition to the hormones' effects on desire, the dryness of the vagina can make sex painful, which can affect a woman's sex drive. The ability to become aroused may also suffer, and some women experience difficulty with orgasm. Some women become less interested in sex because of negative self-esteem related to body image or aging.

As many as half of all women have some drop in sexual desire after menopause.

The good news is that, typically, women who had satisfactory sexual intimacy before menopause continue through perimenopause and beyond. Some women report greater interest in sex after menopause, because the fear of pregnancy is gone, and children are often out of the house.

HAIR LOSS/UNWANTED HAIR

Hair problems are a troublesome symptom for many perimeno-pausal/menopausal women. It's estimated that half of all women have some thinning and hair loss before age fifty, including:

- Thinning of hair from the head or body
- Loss of hair from the head or body
- Receding male-pattern hair loss at the temples
  (known as androgenic alopecia)

The hair loss is most often due to changes in the estrogen/testosterone balance.

While hair loss is a concern, these imbalances can result in hair growing in places where it's not wanted, such as the chin, upper lip, chest, and abdomen.

SKIN CHANGES

As estrogen levels drop, collagen, which gives skin its strength and elasticity, is reduced. Less collagen makes skin thinner, more fragile, and drier, and wrinkles become more prominent. Increasing dryness can also make skin look older and more wrinkled. The layer of fat under the skin tends to thin, which can make wrinkles more visible.

Many women report developing thin vertical wrinkles above the lips, as well as thinning and drying of the lips themselves.

The fluctuations in hormones can also trigger adult-onset acne.

FORMICATION/ITCHINESS/TINGLING SENSATIONS

A symptom some women experience during perimenopause/menopause is called formication, or strange sensations in the skin.

Formication is described as a feeling that resembles insects crawling on or under the skin. Some people describe it as an itchy or even "tingly" sensation.

BONE LOSS

As estrogen declines, women lose bone more quickly than they replace it, resulting in a more rapid loss of bone density.

The optimal bone density for women is usually seen when they are twenty-five to thirty years old. After age thirty, bone density begins to drop, at a rate of less than 1 percent per year. During perimenopause, the bone density loss steps up to as much as 3 percent each year. After menopause, the rate steadies at about 2 percent per year.

Reduced bone mineral density increases the risk of osteoporosis, a disease that weakens bones and increases the risk of disabling or even fatal fractures.

According to the National Osteoporosis Foundation (NOF), osteoporosis is a major public health threat for more than half the population of people fifty years of age and older. According to the NOF, some 10 million individuals already have osteoporosis, and 34 million more are estimated to have low bone mineral density, placing them at increased risk for osteoporosis.

ELEVATED CHOLESTEROL LEVELS

As estrogen levels drop, some women have an increase in the levels of low-density lipoprotein (LDL) cholesterol—known as "bad" cholesterol—as well as the total cholesterol level. At the same time, as we age, levels of high-density lipoprotein (HDL) cholesterol—the "good" cholesterol—tend to drop.

The combination of increasing "bad" cholesterol and dropping "good" cholesterol increases the risk of heart disease.

FATIGUE/LACK OF ENERGY

Fatigue/lack of energy is a symptom that many women associate with perimenopause and menopause.

Some women have a higher level of exhaustion, in general, or need somewhat more sleep in order to feel refreshed. Other women report what's known as "crashing fatigue," which is rapid onset of deep and overwhelming exhaustion that is not related to exertion, sleep, or exercise.

While there is no direct scientific link that says "menopause causes fatigue" or "low estrogen causes fatigue," there are many mechanisms that may be at play. Progesterone is a relaxant, and low progesterone levels in perimenopause and menopause may contribute to anxiety and difficulty sleeping. Other sleep disturbances in perimenopause/menopause can lead to daily fatigue. Also, the adrenal slowdown that can sometimes accompany sex hormone fluctuations can contribute to fatigue.

ACHES AND PAINS

Body aches and pains, along with sore joints, backaches, leg cramps, and muscle tension, are all symptoms that appear to increase in women during perimenopause and menopause. Interestingly, among Japanese women, shoulder stiffness is considered the most severe menopausal complaint and overshadows even hot flashes.

GASTROINTESTINAL/ DIGESTIVE DISTURBANCES

Some women going through perimenopause and menopause report an increase in gastrointestinal and digestive symptoms, including heartburn, indigestion, flatulence, gas pains, nausea, food intolerances, constipation, and bloating/water retention.

DRYNESS

With the drop of estrogen, some women experience dryness not only in the vaginal area, but also in the eyes and mouth. Dry eyes can cause excessive watering, stinging, burning, grittiness, scratchiness, and a sensation that something is in the eye. Dry mouth can contribute to gum problems like gingivitis, increased bleeding, bad breath, a burning tongue, burning feeling in the roof of the mouth, bad taste in the mouth, a change in breath odor, and an increase in dental cavities.

BREAST CHANGES

Menopause may cause changes in the breasts, and women report not only breast tenderness and an increase in lumpy and fibrocystic breasts, but also shrinking, sagging, and reduced firmness.

During perimenopause and menopause, breasts tend to lose muscle and gain fat, which contributes to the sagging.

HEART-RELATED PROBLEMS

During perimenopause and menopause, some women experience heart-related symptoms, including periods of rapid heartbeat, heart palpitations, and an irregular heartbeat, often accompanying hot flashes. While these uncomfortable symptoms are often harmless, women experiencing any heart irregularities need to be evaluated by a doctor before assuming the symptoms are due to perimenopause.

During perimenopause/menopause, women also face an increased risk of heart disease. It's not clear how much of this risk is due to aging, lifestyle, diet, and exercise and how much is caused by the hormonal changes that occur at the time of menopause. But we know that estrogen plays a role, because women who undergo premature menopause or have their ovaries removed surgically at an early age are also at an increased risk of heart disease.

CONCENTRATION AND MEMORY PROBLEMS

According to the North American Menopause Society, 62 percent of women complain of difficulty concentrating, forgetting things more easily, difficulty multitasking, and memory lapses during perimenopause and menopause. Some women refer to it as "brain fog" or "cotton brain." The concentration and memory issues may be due to disrupted sleep and fatigue, but some experts speculate that, because the brain has hundreds of estrogen receptors, a drop in estrogen levels may negatively affect brain function.

HEADACHES/MIGRAINES

Some women who have suffered migraines or chronic headaches report that in perimenopause/menopause, the headaches decrease or even disappear. At the same time, other women report an increase in chronic headaches or migraines.

According to headache and migraine disease expert Teri Robert:

Hormonal fluctuations are frequently a migraine trigger for women. Menopause can be a confusing and frustrating time for women with migraines. Women are often told that their migraines will stop after menopause, but this is not necessarily true. Women for whom monthly hormonal fluctuations have been a lifelong migraine trigger may indeed experience far fewer migraines during and after menopause, but they may also experience more migraines.

OTHER SYMPTOMS

Other symptoms that are more common in perimenopausal and menopausal women, and that may be related to fluctuating hormones, are

- Dizziness, light-headedness, losing your balance
- Changes in body odor
- Changes in foot odor
- Dry, brittle fingernails
- Tinnitus (a ringing, buzzing, or whooshing sound in the ears)
- Varicose veins

chapter 4

Diagnosing and Treating
THYROID PROBLEMS

You can't teach an old dogma new tricks.

—*Dorothy Parker*

Diagnosis of any thyroid problem can include self-checks, but a reliable diagnosis requires a thorough clinical examination by a medical practitioner and a detailed review of the patient's medical history and symptoms, as well as appropriate blood and imaging tests.

Self-Checks

Evaluating your thyroid can start with some self-checks. As with breast self-exams, although self-checks may help you identify a problem, they are not conclusive, and you always need a doctor's evaluation to rule out any sort of thyroid condition.

THE THYROID NECK CHECK

You can perform a simple, at-home self-test to potentially detect some thyroid abnormalities. To do this "thyroid neck check," hold a mirror so that you can see the thyroid area in the neck, just below the Adam's apple and above the collarbone. Tip your head back while keeping this view of your neck and thyroid area visible in the mirror. Take a drink of water and swallow. As you swallow, look at your neck. Watch carefully for any bulges, enlargement, protrusions, or unusual appearances in this area. Repeat this process several times. If you see anything that appears unusual, consult your doctor right away. You may have a goiter (an enlarged thyroid) or a thyroid nodule, and your thyroid should be evaluated. (Be sure you don't get your Adam's apple confused with your thyroid gland. The Adam's apple is at the front of your neck; the thyroid is farther down and closer to your collarbone.)

BASAL BODY TEMPERATURE TEST

It's known that thyroid hormones have a direct effect on the basal, or resting, metabolic rate. And while hypothermia, or lowered body temperature, is a medically accepted symptom of hypothyroidism, the use of basal body temperature (BBT) as a diagnostic tool is quite controversial. The late Broda Barnes, MD, made the public more widely aware of the use of axillary (underarm) BBT as a diagnostic tool for hypothyroidism. It is a monitoring method still used by some complementary and alternative practitioners, but most practitioners suggest that, although regularly low body temperature may suggest a thyroid problem, it is not evidence of it.

To measure your own BBT, use an oral glass/mercury thermometer or a special BBT thermometer available at some pharmacies. For a glass thermometer, shake it down before going to bed, and leave it close by and within reach. As soon as you awake, with minimal movement, put the thermometer in your armpit, next to the skin, and leave it there for ten minutes. Record the readings for three to five consecutive days. Women who still have their menstrual period should not test on the first four days of their period but can begin on day 5. If the temperature regularly falls below the range of 97.8 to 98.2 degrees Fahrenheit, this may point to a possible hypothyroidism condition.

IODINE PATCH TEST

Some practitioners and alternative health resources recommend testing for a potential thyroid problem by putting a patch of iodine on the skin of the arm and seeing if it disappears, and if so, how quickly. (The idea is that if it disappears quickly, the body must be deficient in iodine and suffering from hypothyroidism.) Most holistic practitioners I've surveyed, though, say that they do not use the iodine skin test, since the only thing this test is measuring is how rapidly iodine evaporates. It appears to have nothing to do with thyroid function.

The Clinical Thyroid Examination

Diagnosis of thyroid problems should always include a thorough clinical examination by a physician. The following is a summary of the components of a clinical thyroid exam.

Hands-on examination of the thyroid
The doctor should feel your neck (or palpate) for thyroid enlargement, nodules, and masses. Your doctor will look and feel for goiter, which is an enlargement of the thyroid, as well as nodules or lumps in your thyroid. He or she will also be looking for "thrill" on palpation; this is when the practitioner can "feel" increased blood flow in the thyroid.

Stethoscope examination of the thyroid
The doctor should listen to your thyroid using a stethoscope. He or she should listen for what is known as bruit, the sound of increased blood flow in the thyroid.

Reflex check
The doctor should check your reflexes. Hyperresponsive reflexes can be a sign of hyperthyroidism, and slow reflexes may point to hypothyroidism.

Heart and blood pressure check

Your blood pressure should be checked. Very high or very low blood pressure can be a sign of thyroid problems. Other heart-related issues the doctor should look for are:

- Fast heart rate, known as atypical sinus rhythm or sinus tachycardia: a fast but regular heartbeat over one hundred beats per minute (normal heart rate is 70 to 80 beats per minute)—or bradycardia, a very slow heart rate (under 60 beats per minute in a nonathlete)

- Ventricular tachycardia: rapid heartbeat, felt as palpitations and sometimes also pounding

- Atrial fibrillation: the upper chambers of the heart (atria) and the lower chambers (ventricles) aren't functioning properly, with the atria beating faster than the ventricles, causing an inconsistent rhythm

- Mitral valve prolapse: felt as palpitations and heart flutters

Skin and hair examination

Your skin and hair should be examined for visible signs of a thyroid condition, looking specifically for:

- Loss of the outer edge of eyebrow hair
- Hair loss on the head or body
- Yellowish, jaundiced cast to the skin
- Warm, moist hands and palms
- Hives
- Lesions on the shins (pretibial myxedema/dermopathy)
- Blisterlike bumps on the forehead and face (known as miliaria bumps)

- Onycholysis (separation from the underlying nail bed; also called Plummer's nails)
- Swollen fingertips (acropachy)

Eye examination

Your eyes should be evaluated, and your doctor should be looking for the following possible signs of a thyroid problem:

- Bulging or protruding eyes
- Red, inflamed, and/or bloodshot eyes
- Dry eyes
- Watery eyes
- Stare in the eyes, with retraction of the upper eyelids
- Infrequent blinking
- "Lid lag" (when the upper eyelid doesn't smoothly follow downward movements of the eyes when you look down and instead remains open a bit too long)
- Swelling or puffiness of the eyelids
- Twitching or a tic in the eyes
- Uneven motion of the upper eyelid
- Uneven pupil dilation in dim light
- Tremor of closed eyelids

Other clinical signs your practitioner will look for are

- Tremors
- Shaky hands
- Hyperkinetic movements (for example, table drumming, tapping feet, or jerky movements)
- Enlarged lymph nodes
- A dull facial expression
- Slow movement
- Slow speech

- Hoarseness of voice
- Edema (swelling) of the hands and/or feet

Thyroid Blood Tests

There are several different blood tests that are typically used to diagnose a thyroid condition.

An important note: In some cases, I've included normal ranges and values associated with different tests, but keep in mind that normal ranges can vary from lab to lab and may be expressed quite differently in various countries. Be sure to get a printout of your lab test results, along with information from the lab and your practitioner on what the reference range is for each test (most lab reports will provide this along with the results), so that you can review where your tests fall according to your particular lab.

THYROID-STIMULATING HORMONE

Most doctors rely on the thyroid-stimulating hormone (TSH) test to diagnose an overactive or underactive thyroid. The TSH test measures the amount of TSH in your bloodstream. (The test is sometimes called the thyrotropin–stimulating hormone test.)

When the pituitary detects that there isn't enough circulating thyroid hormone, TSH is released. TSH is considered a messenger that says to the thyroid, "Produce more hormone." So the TSH level goes up when you don't have enough thyroid hormone. A higher TSH level indicates low thyroid hormone production, or hypothyroidism. Conversely, in hyperthyroidism, too much thyroid hormone is circulating, and the TSH level drops.

The TSH level typically remains in what is called the normal reference range when the thyroid gland is healthy and functioning normally.

You'll need to know what the normal values are for the lab where your doctor sends your blood tests because "normal" varies from lab to lab. What is considered a normal thyroid range is in tremendous flux right now. Since the 1980s in North America, the "normal" TSH range has been from about 0.3 to 0.5 at the bottom end, to a high end of from 5.0 to 6.0. At the lab where they sent my blood tests, for example, a TSH level of over 5.5 is considered hypothyroid, and under 0.5 was hyperthyroid. Anywhere in between is considered "normal," or euthyroid.

Values below the low end of the normal TSH range usually indicate hyperthyroidism. In more severe hyperthyroidism, this level may even be undetectable, or 0. Nonexistent or nearly undetectable TSH levels are also referred to as "suppressed" levels. The lower the TSH, the more suppressed the thyroid is considered to be, and the more hyperthyroid you may be.

Values above the top of the normal range can indicate hypothyroidism, an underactive thyroid. The higher the number, the more hypothyroid/underactive your thyroid is considered to be.

In November 2002, the National Academy of Clinical Biochemistry (NACB), part of the American Association for Clinical Chemistry (AACC), issued revised laboratory medicine practice guidelines for the diagnosis and monitoring of thyroid disease. Of particular interest was the following statement in the guidelines:

> More than 95% of rigorously screened normal euthyroid volunteers have serum TSH values between 0.4 and 2.5 mIU/L. . . . A serum TSH result between 0.5 and 2.0 mIU/L is generally considered the therapeutic target for a standard L-T4 replacement dose for primary hypothyroidism.

Based on these findings, in January 2003, the American Association of Clinical Endocrinologists (AACE) made an important announcement:

> Until November 2002, doctors had relied on a normal TSH level ranging from 0.5 to 5.0 to diagnose and treat patients with a thyroid disorder who tested outside the boundaries of that range.

Now AACE encourages doctors to consider treatment for patients who test outside the boundaries of a narrower margin based on a target TSH level of 0.3 to 3.0. AACE believes the new range will result in proper diagnosis for millions of Americans who suffer from a mild thyroid disorder, but have gone untreated until now.

In the years since the original NACB guidelines were released, most laboratories have not yet adopted these new guidelines, and the medical world is still not in complete agreement about changing the guidelines. For example, Labcorp, a lab that is used around the country by many doctors, has a reference range for TSH of 0.45 to 4.50.

This debate continues between practitioners who are using the new range and the labs and doctors using the older, wider range. This means that for patients who test below 0.5 or above 3.0, getting diagnosed for a thyroid condition depends on how up-to-date both the laboratories and the patients' physicians are, and whether they are using the new, narrower standards. The following table summarizes the situation.

TSH Levels

	HYPERTHYROIDISM	"TSH NORMAL"	HYPOTHYROID
	Numbers below range are considered hyperthyroid/ overactive	Reference range (euthyroid)/ thyroid is neither hyperthyroid nor hypothyroid	Numbers above range are considered hypothyroid/ underactive
Former guidelines*	Below 0.5	0.5 to 5.0-6.0	Above 5.0-6.0
New guidelines (per NACB & AACE, as of 2003)	Below 0.3	0.3 to 3.0	Above 3.0

* As of 2009, many laboratories and practitioners are still using these outdated guidelines, and all evidence indicates that this will continue.

AACE, American Association of Clinical Endocrinologists; NACB, National Academy of Clinical Biochemistry; TSH, thyroid-stimulating hormone.

TOTAL THYROXINE (TOTAL T4)

Total T4 measures the total amount of circulating thyroxine (T4) in your blood. Total refers to both the T4 "bound" to protein and the T4 that is free and "unbound." A high value can indicate hyperthyroidism, a low value hypothyroidism. Total T4 levels can be artificially high, however, because pregnancy and estrogen (including the estrogen in hormone therapy and birth control pills) both raise thyroxine-binding globulin (TBG), and TBG elevates total T4 even when the actual levels of T4 circulating in your bloodstream are normal. When bound, thyroid hormone is not available to the cells, so most practitioners prefer to use the free (unbound) T4 test.

FREE THYROXINE (FREE T4)

Free T4 measures the free, unbound thyroxine (T4) levels circulating in your bloodstream. Free T4 is typically lower than normal in hypothyroidism and higher than normal in hyperthyroidism. It is considered a more accurate and reliable test than total T4.

TOTAL TRIIODOTHYRONINE (TOTAL T3)

Total T3 is a measure of the triiodothyronine (T3) bound to protein as well as the T3 that is free and unbound. The total T3 level will typically be lower than normal in hypothyroidism and higher than normal in hyperthyroidism.

FREE TRIIODOTHYRONINE (FREE T3)

Free T3 measures free unbound triiodothyronine in your bloodstream. Again, the free T3 levels are considered more accurate than the total in the case of T3.

THYROGLOBULIN/THYROXINE-BINDING GLOBULIN

Thyroglobulin, also known as thyroxine-binding globulin, or TBG, is a protein produced by the thyroid primarily when it is injured or inflamed due to thyroiditis or cancer. The normal thyroid produces low or no thyroglobulin, so undetectable thyroglobulin levels usually mean normal thyroid function. But when TBG is leaking into the bloodstream and becomes detectable, it indicates some sort of thyroid abnormality. Thyroglobulin is typically elevated in Graves' disease, thyroiditis, and thyroid cancer.

THYROTROPIN-RELEASING HORMONE

The thyrotropin-releasing hormone (TRH) test is a "stimulation" or "challenge" test, rather than a measure of circulating hormones. It's much like a three-hour glucose tolerance test used to diagnose diabetes rather than a fasting glucose level test. The TRH test is considered particularly good for detecting subtle underactive thyroid problems. The time and cost involved in the test, as well as the difficulty getting the drugs needed to perform the test, however, have made it all but impossible to get from most physicians. It is therefore rarely used.

REVERSE T3

When the body is under stress, instead of converting T4 into T3 (the active form of thyroid hormone that works at the cellular level), it conserves energy by making an inactive form of T3 known as reverse T3 (RT3). Some practitioners believe that even when stress is relieved, people continue to manufacture RT3 instead of active T3. This in turn creates a thyroid problem at the cellular level, even though TSH lab values may well be normal. The values of RT3 tests are controversial, but this test has become somewhat more popular with open-minded doctors who are looking to assess a person's full range of thyroid function.

THYROID PEROXIDASE ANTIBODIES/ANTITHYROID
PEROXIDASE ANTIBODIES

One of the most common thyroid antibody blood tests is thyroid peroxidase (TPO) antibodies, also known as antithyroid peroxidase, or anti-TPO, antibodies. This test is often done as a first step in diagnosing autoimmune thyroid disease. TPO antibodies attack thyroid peroxidase, an enzyme that plays a part in the conversion of T4 to T3. They can indicate that the thyroid tissue is being destroyed, such as in Hashimoto's disease and in some other types of thyroiditis, such as postpartum thyroiditis. TPO antibodies are detectable in approximately 95 percent of patients with Hashimoto's thyroiditis. It's thought that among patients with Graves' disease, 50 to 85 percent will test positive for these antibodies.

ANTITHYROID MICROSOMAL ANTIBODIES

In some cases, antithyroid microsomal antibodies are measured, but the TPO antibody test is now considered more state of the art and has replaced this test in part. The level of antithyroid microsomal antibodies is typically elevated in Hashimoto's thyroiditis. It's thought that as much as 80 percent of Hashimoto's patients have elevated levels of these antibodies.

THYROGLOBULIN ANTIBODIES/
ANTITHYROGLOBULIN ANTIBODIES

Testing for thyroglobulin antibodies (also called antithyroglobulin antibodies) is common. Thyroglobulin antibodies are positive in about 60 percent of Hashimoto's patients and 30 percent of Graves' patients.

THYROID STIMULATING HORMONE RECEPTOR ANTIBODIES

TSH receptor antibodies are seen in most patients with a history of or who currently have Graves' disease. They may be:

* Stimulatory, in which case they cause hyperthyroidism (TSH-stimulating antibodies)
* Blocking, in which case they prevent TSH from binding to the cell receptor and cause hypothyroidism (TSH receptor blocking antibodies)
* Binding, in which case they interfere with the activity of TSH at the cell receptor

Patients with Graves' disease tend to test positive for stimulatory TSH receptor antibodies, and patients with Hashimoto's disease tend to test positive for blocking TSH receptor antibodies.

THYROID-STIMULATING IMMUNOGLOBULINS

Thyroid-stimulating immunoglobulins (TSIs) can be detected in the majority of patients with Graves' disease. Their presence is considered diagnostic. The higher the levels, the more active the Graves' disease is thought to be. The absence of these antibodies does not, however, mean that you don't have Graves' disease. Some people with autoimmune hypothyroidism also have TSIs, and this can cause periodic transient hyperthyroid episodes.

THYROID IMAGING TESTS

Several types of imaging and evaluation tests are used to make a conclusive diagnosis of thyroid disease.

Nuclear Scan/Radioactive Iodine Uptake

Radioactive iodine uptake (RAI-U) is used to help differentiate Graves' disease, toxic multinodular goiter, and thyroiditis. In this test, a small dose of radioactive iodine 123 is administered as a pill. Several hours later, the amount of iodine in your system is measured, accompanied by an x-ray that views how iodine is concentrated in your thyroid.

An overactive thyroid usually takes up higher amounts of iodine than normal, and that uptake is visible on the x-ray. A thyroid that takes up iodine is considered "hot," or overactive; an underactive thyroid is "cold."

In Graves' disease, RAI-U is elevated, and you can see that the entire gland becomes hot. (In contrast, in Hashimoto's thyroiditis, the uptake is usually low, with patchy hot spots in the gland.) If you have thyroid nodules, RAI-U can show them and whether they are hot. Hot nodules may overproduce thyroid hormone, but they are rarely cancerous. Cold nodules (nodules that do not take up iodine) can be cancerous and require further follow-up. An estimated 10 to 20 percent of cold nodules are cancerous.

Computed Tomography Scan

A computed tomography (CT) scan—or "cat" scan—is a specialized imaging technique that can be used to evaluate the thyroid. The scan cannot detect smaller nodules, but it can diagnose a goiter or larger nodules.

Magnetic Resonance Imaging

Magnetic resonance imaging (MRI) is done when the size and shape of the thyroid need to be evaluated. MRI can't tell anything about how your thyroid is functioning—that is, whether it is hyperthyroid or hypothyroid—but it can detect enlargement and may be done along with blood tests. It is sometimes preferable to x-rays or CT scans because it doesn't require any injection of contrast dye and doesn't require to radiation.

Thyroid Ultrasound

Ultrasound of the thyroid is done to evaluate nodules, lumps, and enlargement of the gland. It also can determine whether a nodule is a fluid-filled cyst or a mass of solid tissue. Ultrasound cannot tell whether a nodule or lump is benign or malignant, however.

Needle Biopsy/Fine Needle Aspiration

Needle biopsy or fine needle aspiration (FNA) helps to evaluate suspicious lumps or cold nodules. In a needle biopsy, a thin needle is inserted directly into the lump, and some cells are withdrawn and evaluated. In some cases, ultrasound is used to help guide the needle into the correct position. Pathology assessment of the cells can often reveal Hashimoto's thyroiditis, as well as cancerous cells. Definitive information is available in approximately 75 percent of nodules biopsied.

Diagnosing a Thyroid Problem

Based on the results of the patient history, review of symptoms, clinical examination, and blood and imaging tests, doctors should be able to make an accurate diagnosis.

DIAGNOSING HYPOTHYROIDISM

To diagnose hypothyroidism, in addition to the history, symptoms, and clinical examination, conventional doctors consider the TSH test results. A TSH level above the reference range is considered hypothyroid and will be flagged as high on test results. Remember, however, that there is controversy over the reference range, with some groups recommending the new range of 0.3 to 3.0, and many labs and doctors still using the old range of 0.5 to around 5.5.

Other blood tests that are typically done to help diagnose hypothyroidism are

- Free T4 (free thyroxine): a low level along with an elevated TSH may indicate hypothyroidism.
- Free T3 (free triiodothyronine): a low level along with an elevated TSH may indicate hypothyroidism.

DIAGNOSING HASHIMOTO'S THYROIDITIS

Hashimoto's thyroiditis is the most common cause of hypothyroidism. The characteristic Hashimoto's thyroiditis patient would have high or high-normal TSH values and low or low-normal free T3 and free T4 levels. The greatest distinguishing feature for Hashimoto's is a high concentration of thyroid autoantibodies, particularly anti-TPO antibodies. (Some patients have elevated antibody levels for months or even years before the TSH level changes. But elevated antibodies can cause symptoms, and there is some evidence that treating elevated antibodies with a low dose of thyroid hormone medication may help reduce antibodies and prevent progression to overt hypothyroidism.)

Occasionally, FNA of thyroid nodules/lumps will reveal evidence of Hashimoto's disease, but FNA typically is not done just to diagnose Hashimoto's disease.

DIAGNOSING HYPERTHYROIDISM

A diagnosis of hyperthyroidism is usually made by means of a TSH test. Levels below 0.3 to 0.5 may be considered hyperthyroid.

Other blood tests that may be done to help diagnose hyperthyroidism are

- **Free T4:** a high level along with a low TSH may indicate hyperthyroidism.
- **Free T3:** a high level along with a low TSH may indicate hyperthyroidism.

DIAGNOSING GRAVES' DISEASE

In addition to hyperthyroid TSH levels (typically, a TSH level below 0.3) and high-normal or high levels of free T4 and free T3, the levels of TSH antibodies and TSI may be measured to diagnose Graves' disease, the autoimmune condition that frequently causes hyperthyroidism.

A radioactive picture of the thyroid, made by ingesting a small amount of radioactive iodine, may also be taken to see if the gland is overactive. This overactivity is a hallmark of Graves' disease.

DIAGNOSING GOITER

Several steps can be involved in diagnosing the enlarged thyroid known as goiter:

- Examining and observing the neck enlargement
- A blood test to determine if the thyroid is producing irregular amounts of thyroid hormone
- Antibodies testing to confirm that autoimmune disease may be the cause of the goiter

- An ultrasound test to evaluate the size of the enlarged thyroid
- A radioactive thyroid scan to produce an image of the thyroid and provide visual information about the nature of the thyroid enlargement

DIAGNOSING THYROID NODULES

Nodules are usually evaluated by

- A blood test, to determine whether a nodule is producing thyroid hormone
- A radioactive thyroid scan, which looks at the reaction of the nodule to small amounts of radioactive material
- An ultrasound of the thyroid to determine whether the nodule is solid or fluid-filled
- FNA or needle biopsy of the nodule to evaluate whether it is cancerous

DIAGNOSING THYROID CANCER

The main diagnostic procedure for suspected thyroid cancer is FNA of the thyroid nodule. In FNA, a needle is inserted into the nodules or lumps. Fluid and cells are removed from various parts of the nodules, and these samples are then evaluated. Sometimes FNA is done with an ultrasound to help guide the needle into nodules that are too small to be felt. Between 60 and 80 percent of FNA tests show that the nodule is benign. Only about one of twenty FNA tests reveals cancer. The remainder of the cases are classified as suspicious, and frequently a surgical biopsy is needed in order to rule out or diagnose cancer.

Challenges to Getting Properly Diagnosed

While it's common for doctors to say that thyroid disease is easy to diagnose and easy to treat, the reality is that diagnosis can be complicated. Many doctors don't recognize thyroid symptoms, so patients mistakenly are prescribed estrogen, antidepressants, weight loss drugs, or cholesterol medications instead of given a thyroid test. Once thyroid problems are suspected, some doctors will perform only a TSH test, then base their diagnosis only on that result. This narrow approach misses patients who otherwise would be diagnosed by a thorough thyroid evaluation, such as one that takes into account clinical examination, review of symptoms, a thorough family and personal history, and other blood work and imaging tests as needed.

UNINFORMED DOCTORS

Surprisingly in this day and age, there are still practitioners who believe that they can simply look at a patient, or feel his or her neck, and rule out thyroid disease. Looking at the patient and feeling the thyroid for enlargement and lumps are only a small part of a clinical thyroid examination. As noted, a thorough clinical thyroid exam must also include a blood pressure and pulse check, weight check, evaluation of reflexes, and careful evaluation of clinical thyroid signs, such as loss of outer eyebrow hair, swelling in face and limbs, unusual skin patches, and other skin and hair disturbances. The doctor should then consider the findings, in addition to blood work and medical history, to make a diagnosis. If you are seeing a doctor who thinks he or she can rule out thyroid disease based on looking at you or feeling your thyroid, get another doctor.

"BY THE NUMBERS" DIAGNOSIS

Today's conventional thyroid treatment tends to focus on blood test results to the exclusion of how patients feel. One prominent endocrinologist even declared that thyroid patients who had "normal" TSH levels after treatment but who continued to have debilitating symptoms were likely suffering from mental illness. This has to change. Practicing medicine is a lot more than just reading numbers off a chart.

Some doctors believe that, even in the face of obvious thyroid signs and symptoms, unless the numbers clearly demonstrate a problem, they won't make a thyroid diagnosis. Holistic practitioner Dr. Jocelyne Eberstein has a problem with this approach:

> Too many doctors just look at the numbers. They don't even look up from their paper to see the patient is losing hair, constipated, and suffering from other symptoms. Practitioners aren't looking, they aren't touching.

It's important to note that there is a major disagreement between those practitioners who believe that blood tests must be abnormal in order to diagnose thyroid disease and justify treatment and those who feel that blood tests are only a small part of the picture. The more holistic, integrative doctors typically consider a patient's complete situation—including family history, personal history, symptoms, clinical examination, and blood tests—rather than relying only on blood test results.

Getting a proper diagnosis sometimes means you will need to remind your doctor that you are a patient, not a lab value. Spell out your symptoms and family history, insist on a thorough thyroid evaluation, and be sure that the doctor's goal is resolving symptoms, not just looking at test results. When necessary, abandon a conservative, less innovative physician, and switch to one who will take a big picture view of thyroid diagnosis.

USEFULNESS OF THE TSH TEST

There are many practitioners who run the TSH—and only the TSH test—to diagnose and manage thyroid conditions. But some doctors feel that the TSH test alone is simply not very useful. Dr. Jocelyne Eberstein wonders about the usefulness of the test.

> Why measure a stimulating hormone when you're trying to check a hormone level? It's like checking a man's luteinizing hormone if you're trying to evaluate his testosterone levels. This is why we need to actually check free T3 and free T4.

Again, some practitioners tend to rely on the TSH as the only test they need to diagnose and treat thyroid conditions. But to get a proper diagnosis, you may need to switch to a practitioner who will consider other tests (like free T4, free T3, and antibodies tests), as well as your clinical signs, symptoms, and history.

QUALITY/RELIABILITY OF THE TSH TEST

While many doctors assume that the TSH test is accurate, some have concerns about the reliability of the TSH test and feel it's unwise to rely on this test alone for diagnosis and management.

Dr. Richard Shames, a noted thyroid practitioner and author of a number of books on thyroid disease, has found that many practitioners take TSH blood samples but allow those samples to sit for many hours before they are collected and shipped to the laboratory for analysis. Says Dr. Shames:

> These samples are supposed to be cooled and packed in ice. But often they're not. Or they have been sitting around for hours before even traveling to the lab. The TSH in the sample can degrade in transit. A TSH that might have been measured at a 6.0 or 7.0 can degrade so that by the time it's measured, it actually ends up in the normal range.

Dr. Shames has seen situations where patients were being properly managed on thyroid medication and symptoms were relieved, then had a TSH test that showed that their TSH was too low. Says Dr. Shames:

> It didn't make sense. But when we retested, it turned out that their TSH was fine, and no dosage change was needed. But when doctors trust the TSH and don't realize that some of these samples are degraded, patients may not get proper treatment.

There is also the issue of time of day affecting the TSH level. The highest TSH level is typically obtained from a fasting blood test administered first thing in the morning. One study found that TSH levels drop—by an average of 26 percent—when compared with the early morning level. This means that as many as 6 percent of patients would be reclassified from hypothyroid levels to "normal" TSH.

A patient who might have a high or high-normal TSH if tested earlier in the day could have a normal TSH if tested later in the day.

Getting a proper diagnosis sometimes means you will need to be careful when and where you have your blood work done and ask about how the sample will be stored before it's sent to the lab for analysis. Given the significant questions about the TSH reliability overall, you may also need to see a physician who does not base his or her entire diagnosis on this test alone.

INTERPRETATION OF THE TSH TEST

Many practitioners consider the TSH test the gold standard for diagnosing thyroid disease. Unfortunately, as noted, there is still a major disconnect in the medical community over how to interpret the results of that test. Progressive practitioners tend to use the narrower, more recent range of 0.3 to 3.0, while others use the older reference range of 0.5 to 5.5. You could have a list of thyroid symptoms, a family history, and clinical signs of a thyroid condition, yet if your TSH test result came back at 4.9, one doctor might tell you your thyroid is normal, and another might tell you are hypothyroid. So much for the gold standard.

It's estimated that if the new narrow range were adopted nationally, 30 million more people would be considered as having thyroid disease. But with the ongoing disagreement, the vast majority of these people remain in an undiagnosed limbo.

If you are told that your thyroid test is "normal," you need to first find out the exact numbers and what range the doctor is using to define normal. Better yet, ask when you're scheduling your appointment what range the doctor uses. And if you fall into the limbo of a

TSH level between 3.0 and 5.5 and are told you're normal, get another opinion from a more up-to-date practitioner.

FEAR OF OSTEOPOROSIS

Some practitioners have a fear that treating mild or borderline hypothyroidism will increase a woman's risk of osteoporosis. This fear is based on research that has shown that extended periods of hyperthyroidism, in particular, extremely low, suppressed TSH levels, can be a risk factor for osteoporosis. There are also several inconclusive studies that suggest that long-term treatment of hypothyroidism may increase the risk of osteoporosis. At the same time, there are a number of other studies that show that thyroid treatment does not increase the risk of osteoporosis.

Some doctors, unfortunately, employ faulty logic and decide if a very low TSH level poses a risk, and treatment *might* pose a risk, then keeping perimenopausal and menopausal hypothyroid women at higher levels will avoid the risk.

An important review looked at sixty-three English-language studies of the thyroid–osteoporosis connection that were published from 1990 to 2001. Of the studies reviewed, levothyroxine was shown to have no overall effect in thirty-one studies, partial positive and/or partial negative effects were reported in twenty-three studies, only nine studies showed overall negative effects, and three studies reported no effects. Ultimately, this metareview found no association between the duration of levothyroxine therapy and an associated reduction of bone mineral density.

DOCTORS WHO WON'T ORDER TESTS/HMOS AND INSURANCE COMPANIES THAT WON'T COVER TESTS

Sometimes you will come up against a doctor who, for a number of reasons, simply refuses to order blood tests for your thyroid treatment. It may be a doctor who is trying to control costs (often in an HMO environment) or who has decided that, simply by looking at you, he or she can "tell" that you don't have a thyroid condition and therefore don't need testing. Or a doctor could become territorial and refuse to run thyroid tests unless it was his idea. (Ridiculous, I know, but far more common than you think.)

In some cases, HMOs and insurance companies simply won't approve thyroid tests or will only approve TSH tests.

In these circumstances, you have several options.

1. Put together a detailed checklist of your risks and symptoms (you can print out detailed Risks and Symptoms checklists for Thyroid Disease and Perimenopause/Menopause from my Web site at www.menopausethyroid.com). Bring this checklist with you to your next doctor's appointment and politely ask the doctor to sign and date the checklist, adding a note indicating that he or she has reviewed the checklist and refused to do thyroid tests for you. (Typically, most doctors would rather order the tests than go on the record as having refused them.)

2. You can appeal to the ombudsman or patient representative of your HMO or insurance company, asking them to reconsider covering the costs of the tests. Again, send a copy of your checklist or a memo summarizing your risks and symptoms to support your complaint.

3. You can bypass your physician, HMO, or insurance company and order your own blood tests. In most states (except New York, New Jersey, and Rhode Island, which have laws preventing patients from ordering their own medical tests) you can order your own blood tests, including TSH, free T4, free T3, thyroid antibodies— and hundreds of other tests—using a service like MyMedLab or ZRT Labs. By ordering and paying for your own tests, you are able to get them at very low cost, thanks to group purchasing power and a lack of doctor's office markups. The cost is less than you would pay going directly to the lab and is sometimes even less

expensive than your insurance co-pay for these tests at full-price plus markup. While you should always work with a physician for interpretation of any unusual results, proper diagnosis, and safe treatment of any problems, self-testing can be a helpful first step. It is also an affordable option if your doctor, HMO, or insurance company is putting up unnecessary impediments to testing or if you are unable to get costs reimbursed.

Thyroid Treatments

HYPERTHYROIDISM/OVERACTIVE THYROID: THYROTOXICOSIS

If you are in the United States, the treatment most often recommended for hyperthyroidism and Graves' disease is radioactive iodine (RAI), sometimes referred to as ablation therapy or chemical ablation. This involves taking a liquid or pill form of radioactive iodine, which is then absorbed by the thyroid. The RAI disables the thyroid, usually permanently. Most patients who have RAI treatment develop the opposite condition—hypothyroidism—and require thyroid hormone replacement for life. Some physicians in the United States take a less drastic approach and prescribe antithyroid drugs such as propylthiouracil (PTU) and methimazole (brand names Tapazole and Carbimazole), along with beta blockers like propanolol or atenolol, to calm down the thyroid, the immune system, and the heart rate/blood pressure. This approach is based on the chance of remission of hyperthyroidism and disease, which occurs in up to 30 percent of patients. (Interestingly, antithyroid drugs are the first choice in treatment for doctors outside the United States.) In rarer cases in the United States, and more commonly outside the United States, surgery to remove the thyroid may be advised. Holistic and integrative treatments prior to RAI or surgery focus on complementing antithyroid drug approaches with foods, supplements, and herbs that can slow down the thyroid but have few side effects. Some patients have also had success with calming and rebalancing the immune system through nutrition, herbs, supplements, movement therapy such as yoga, and energy work. Ultimately, most people with Graves' disease and hyperthyroidism do end up hypothyroid for life as a result of RAI or surgery.

My book *Living Well with Graves' Disease and Hyperthyroidism* provides more in-depth information on the various treatment options, both conventional and holistic, and also details a holistic and integrative protocol for Graves' disease and overactive thyroid problems.

GOITER/ENLARGEMENT

Goiter can be due to an autoimmune condition that triggers an inflamed thyroid, or it can be caused by too much or too little iodine in the diet. In the United States, 10 to 20 percent of goiters are iodine-induced. Treatment for goiter depends on how enlarged the thyroid has become, as well as other symptoms. Treatment can include

- Observation and monitoring, which is typically done if the goiter is not large and is not causing symptoms or thyroid dysfunction

- Iodine supplementation if iodine deficiency is the cause of the goiter

- Medications, including thyroid hormone replacement, which can help shrink the goiter, or aspirin or corticosteroid drugs to minimize thyroid inflammation

- If the goiter is very large, continues to grow despite thyroid hormone therapy, or symptoms continue, or if the goiter is in a dangerous location (that is, pressing against the windpipe or esophagus), or if it is cosmetically unsightly, most doctors will recommend surgery. If the goiter contains any suspicious nodules, that may also be reason for surgery.

NODULES/LUMPS

Benign nodules are often left alone and monitored periodically, assuming they aren't causing serious difficulty. Some will be treated with thyroid hormone replacement to help shrink them, a treatment that is not considered universally effective.

Some emerging treatments, including percutaneous ethanol injections and ultrasound, are being used by cutting-edge practitioners to treat nodules.

Nodules are surgically removed if they are causing difficulties with breathing or swallowing.

Nodules that are considered suspicious, or that show evidence of cancer, are removed along with the thyroid gland itself.

THYROID CANCER

The treatments for thyroid cancer almost always involve surgery to remove the thyroid and cancer. In some cases, lymph node dissection also removes lymph nodes in the neck that contain cancer. RAI treatment is typically given as a follow-up to surgery. Because the thyroid takes up iodine, the radioactive iodine collects in any thyroid tissue remaining in the body and kills the cancer cells. Less commonly, external radiation therapy may be given. Hormone therapy, using thyroid hormone replacement medication, is often included.

Because the entire thyroid is removed as treatment for most thyroid cancers, almost all thyroid cancer survivors end up hypothyroid and need to take thyroid replacement hormone for life. Their thyroid medication needs to be at a high enough dose to ensure that their TSH levels remain low (nearly undetectable, actually) to help prevent a relapse of cancer. Survivors need regular checkups to watch for a reoccurrence.

HASHIMOTO'S DISEASE/THYROIDITIS

Typically, because Hashimoto's disease most often causes hypothyroidism, the conventional approach is simply to treat the hypothyroidism with thyroid hormone replacement medication. Conventional medicine offers no treatment for the autoimmunity of Hashimoto's itself.

Holistic and integrative approaches to Hashimoto's tend to look at healing the underlying autoimmune imbalance, and may include nutritional support for the thyroid (selenium, tyrosine, B vitamins, etc.) and overall support for the immune system.

HYPOTHYROIDISM

The end result for most thyroid patients is hypothyroidism, an underactive thyroid condition that requires thyroid hormone replacement for life.

With the autoimmune disease Hashimoto's thyroiditis, the thyroid typically burns itself out over time, becoming less able to produce thyroid hormone and leaving most patients hypothyroid.

With Graves' disease and hyperthyroidism, most patients in the United States have RAI treatment, which usually leaves them without a functional thyroid. This means they end up hypothyroid, even if they started with an overactive gland.

With thyroid nodules and goiter, surgery may be performed to remove all or part of the thyroid. The end result is frequently hypothyroidism.

For thyroid cancer, almost all patients have their thyroid removed entirely, leaving them completely hypothyroid and reliant on outside thyroid hormone replacement.

So, whatever the thyroid disease or condition, patients are likely to end up hypothyroid in the end, unable to produce sufficient thyroid hormone on their own and requiring thyroid hormone replacement treatment.

Conventional treatment typically involves replacing the missing thyroid hormone, using prescription thyroid hormone replacement drugs. These medications are discussed in the next section. Holistic approaches to an underactive thyroid are also discussed later in this chapter.

Thyroid Medications

LEVOTHYROXINE

The most commonly prescribed thyroid hormone replacement drug is levothyroxine, the generic name for the synthetic form of thyroxine (T4). It is sometimes referred to as l-thyroxine or L-T4, and some endocrinologists also incorrectly call it thyroxine, which is actually the name of the hormone produced in the body.

Most commonly, a levothyroxine drug is prescribed for hypothyroidism due to any cause, as conventional doctors consider it to be the standard treatment for hypothyroidism.

Many doctors will only prescribe levothyroxine for thyroid hormone replacement. The rationale is that people only need the synthetic T4, and the body will convert the T4 in the medication to T3 (triiodothyronine), the active thyroid hormone at the cellular level. Some people with hypothyroidism find that levothyroxine therapy is sufficient treatment for their hypothyroidism.

Many doctors do not recommend generic levothyroxine, preferring brand names instead. This is because the different generic versions of levothyroxine can vary in some cases from 95 to 105 percent of the stated potency, causing symptoms and testing irregularities. (For thyroid cancer survivors, erratic dosing can jeopardize therapy to prevent cancer recurrence.)

The different brand names of levothyroxine are for the most part equivalent in terms of effectiveness. The primary difference between brand names is that each has different fillers, binders, and dyes, and some patients may have allergies to those ingredients. The 50 mcg (microgram) dosage pills from the brand-name levothyroxine manufacturers are typically free of dyes and are more likely to be hypoallergenic.

Levothyroxine came on the market in the late 1950s, without approval from the U.S. Food and Drug Administration (FDA). It was grandfathered in under approval for natural dessicated thyroid, which had been available since the early 1900s. In 1997 the FDA required all levothyroxine drugs to go through the new drug application process and receive formal approval, given concerns over their stability, potency, and reliability. The drugs were to be approved by 2000, but only Unithroid (distributed as a generic by Lannett; formerly manufactured by Jerome Stevens) received approval within the FDA deadline. The other main brands—Levoxyl (Jones Pharma, a subsidiary of King Pharmaceuticals), Levothroid (Forest Pharmaceuticals), and Synthroid (Abbott Laboratories)—were eventually approved.

Synthroid, as a heavily marketed drug for more than four decades, enjoys a high degree of brand loyalty from physicians. Over the years, Synthroid's manufacturer has been a heavy financial supporter of medical meetings and physician education, and has taken many opportunities to get Synthroid's name in front of new and established physicians. As a result, Synthroid is sometimes used by doctors to describe the whole category of "thyroid hormone replacement drugs" (in the same way that the brand name Kleenex has, for example, become synonymous with "tissue" or Xerox with photocopying).

LIOTRIX (THYROLAR)

Thyrolar (Forest Pharmaceuticals) is the brand name for liotrix, a combination of synthetic T4 (levothyroxine) and synthetic T3 (liothyronine). This drug is not very regularly prescribed, but it is preferred by some physicians who wish to provide both T4 and T3 but prefer a synthetic versus natural desiccated thyroid.

It's important to note how to properly store Thyrolar. Thyrolar needs to be kept at a refrigerated temperature between 36 and 46 degrees Fahrenheit (2 to 8 degrees Celsius). This refrigeration will ensure that Thyrolar remains potent and stable. According to the manufacturer's pharmacists, refrigeration will actually help the product maintain optimal potency longer. If you need to travel, however, the product should remain stable for at least a week. So you don't have to go to extraordinary lengths to keep Thyrolar refrigerated while traveling.

LIOTHYRONINE/T3

Liothyronine (brand name Cytomel, distributed by Jones Pharma Inc., a subsidiary of King Pharmaceuticals) is the synthetic form of triiodothyronine (T3), the active thyroid hormone at the cellular level.

Research has shown that some patients feel better with the addition of T3 in some form, so practitioners prescribe a form of liothyronine along with a levothyroxine medication, or natural thyroid medication.

Francesca, who is perimenopausal with a thyroid problem, started going to a new nurse practitioner, who put her on Cytomel. Says Francesca:

My only side effect was a minor headache for two days, which went away with aspirin. The third day I realized I was awake. I woke up in the morning and was "alert" for the first time in years. It didn't take me an hour to drag myself out of bed. I was only taking 5 micrograms of Cytomel and had an immediate result. My body temperature has risen to 98.1 degrees Fahrenheit, and I am noticing little things changing in my body and health.

Liothyronine is also available from compounding pharmacies, who can make it available in regular or time-released capsules.

Dr. Richard Shames has found that T3 can be a helpful addition to a patient's thyroid therapy. Says Dr. Shames:

When it comes to T3, some patients do well on Cytomel, but it seems that some patients do better on time-released T3. It seems that the compounded, time-released form prevents that spike of T3 that you get with Cytomel. For some patients, the time-released T3 provides the necessary gradient that helps to drive the T3 across the cell membrane barrier.

Sometimes thyroid cancer patients preparing for a scan are given Cytomel for several weeks, to help aid with hypothyroidism symptoms that result from withdrawal from other thyroid medication, which is needed for the scan's accuracy.

A controversial form of thyroid treatment for hypothyroidism is T3-only treatment, and few doctors recommend this approach.

NATURAL DESICCATED THYROID

Natural desiccated thyroid is the original form of thyroid hormone replacement that first came into use in the early 1900s. It is thyroid medication derived from the thyroid gland of animals that is dried and measured to ensure proper potency. It contains natural forms of the thyroid hormones T4 and T3, as well as other, lesser known thyroid hormones, such as T2 and T1, the hormone calcitonin, and nutrients typically found in a natural thyroid gland. Decades ago, bovine (cow) thyroid was used, but prescription natural thyroid sold in the United States is currently porcine (pig).

From the early 1900s until the 1950s, natural desiccated thyroid was the only form of thyroid replacement drug available. In the late 1950s/early 1960s, the drug fell out of favor with many endocrinologists, as Synthroid's extensive marketing promoted synthetic thyroid as a better, more "modern" option for thyroid treatment.

Marketing efforts aside, since the 1990s, Armour Thyroid (Forest Pharmaceuticals), along with other brands of natural thyroid, like Nature-Throid and WesThroid (both from Western Research Labs), have been enjoying a resurgence in popularity with increasing numbers of patients and practitioners. These doctors, more often osteopaths, naturopaths, and holistic practitioners, prefer to start their hypothyroid patients on a desiccated thyroid drug, because they believe that since the drug contains a full spectrum of thyroid hormones as well as nutritional cofactors, it more closely mimics the action of human thyroid hormone, and their patients generally respond better.

The top-selling brand of natural thyroid is Armour Thyroid,

bound by microcrystalline cellulose. Westhroid is cornstarch-bound. Nature-Throid is bound with microcrystalline cellulose and is hypoallergenic.

Most endocrinologists and conventional practitioners tend to oppose the use of natural thyroid on principle, primarily based on outdated concerns about potency, or because they are unfamiliar with the current manufacturing processes for desiccated thyroid or how to properly dose these medications.

ANTITHYROID DRUGS

Antithyroid drugs have been in use since the 1940s. They are given to help achieve a remission in hyperthyroidism and its symptoms. One key antithyroid drug is methimazole (brand name Tapazole, distributed by Jones Pharma, a subsidiary of King Pharmaceuticals), sometimes also called thiamazole. This drug is used around the world. Carbimazole (brand name NeoMercazole, made by Nicholas Piramal) is a similar medication that metabolizes to methimazole. It is typically used in the United Kingdom and elsewhere in Europe.

The other main antithyroid drug is propylthiouracil, usually referred to as PTU. PTU is available only as a generic.

Methimazole inhibits the thyroid from using iodine to produce thyroid hormone. PTU has two effects. Not only does it inhibit the thyroid from using iodine to produce thyroid hormone, but it also inhibits T4-to-T3 conversion. PTU has a shorter half-life than methimazole and acts more quickly, so some people see the effects of PTU right away. Also, because PTU blocks T4-to-T3 conversion, it is thought to act faster and may more quickly reduce T3 levels, resolving symptoms more quickly, compared with methimazole. PTU, therefore, is sometimes given in thyroid storm (an emergency of the thyroid) or during severe hyperthyroidism because of its fast-acting characteristics. Because methimazole is longer acting, it is preferred by some doctors and patients because less frequent dosing is required.

THYROTROPIN ALFA/RECOMBINANT TSH

Thyrogen (Genzyme Therapeutics) is the brand name of thyrotropin alfa, also known as recombinant TSH. This drug, given only by injection, is for thyroid cancer patients. When thyroid cancer patients are preparing to have a scan to assess recurrence or leftover cancer cells, they usually need to stop taking thyroid hormone replacement drugs (usually, levothyroxine), in order to improve the accuracy of the scans. Unfortunately, the result of withdrawing thyroid hormone replacement is several weeks to months of hypothyroidism, including side effects such as severe fatigue, weight gain, depression, memory problems, confusion, and constipation. For certain patients, Thyrogen can be injected and will prevent the symptoms of hypothyroidism, without compromising the ability to conduct a scan. A scan using Thyrogen is considered slightly less sensitive than a scan on total withdrawal of all thyroid hormone replacement, so Thyrogen scans are often recommended for long-term survivors and for those who have had a few years of negative tests under conventional hormone withdrawal.

Optimizing Your Thyroid Hormone Replacement Treatment

Because most patients end up hypothyroid, it's important to ensure that your treatment is optimized.

To optimize your treatment, you'll want to consider the following important questions.

IF YOU'RE ON LEVOTHYROXINE, IS IT THE RIGHT BRAND FOR YOU?

Because of their differences in fillers, binders, and dyes, different formulations of levothyroxine may produce different reactions in patients. For example, Synthroid is known to digest very slowly, while Levoxyl is fast-dissolving. Synthroid contains acacia and lactose, which can cause problems in some people who are sensitive.

With a number of FDA-approved brand-name levothyroxine drugs available, you may wish to discuss a change in brand with your physician. Do stick with a brand name, however, and not a generic, to ensure consistency from refill to refill.

DO YOU NEED T3?

Some people do not feel their best without the addition of the active thyroid hormone T3. Usually, the body converts T4 to enough T3, but nutritional deficiencies, toxins, and a variety of other physiological factors may prevent the body from effectively handling that conversion, which can leave you deficient in this most important thyroid hormone. While it's a controversial topic that is under increasing study by various experts, some physicians find that supplemental T3 helps optimize thyroid treatment for some patients. They add T3 in one of several ways:

- Prescribing the T3 drug Cytomel, or a compounded T3 pill, in addition to levothyroxine treatment
- Prescribing the combination synthetic drug Thyrolar, which includes both T4 and T3
- Prescribing natural desiccated thyroid, such as the prescription drug Armour Thyroid, Nature-Throid, or WesThroid, which also has a full array of natural thyroid hormones, including T3

Check with your physician about whether or not supplemental T3 might be helpful for you. But realize that many conventional physicians will not be willing to even discuss T3, much less prescribe it, and you may need to seek a more open-minded practitioner.

WOULD NATURAL THYROID HELP?

Some practitioners find that, in general, their patients do best on natural desiccated thyroid, derived from the thyroid gland of pigs. These products, including Armour, WesThroid, and Nature-Throid, are prescription thyroid drugs that have been in use as long as one hundred years. Many patients who have switched from synthetic to natural thyroid swear by the improvements in health and symptoms they've enjoyed after taking the natural medication.

Keep in mind that many conventional physicians feel that these drugs are "out of date" or hard to regulate or prescribe, and so won't prescribe them.

Jeffersonville, Pennsylvania–based holistic physician Dr. Martin Mulders has changed his own opinion of Armour Thyroid:

> I find that patients generally do better on desiccated thyroid. . . . I use it all the time. Back in the early 1990s, however, I was saying that "Armour Thyroid is hard to regulate," like some doctors say. But I've since learned that it's absolutely not true. In my opinion, doctors who say that it's difficult haven't tried it with their patients.

IS YOUR TREATMENT OPTIMIZED?

Kensington, Maryland–based holistic physician and thyroid patient Adrienne Clamp, MD, believes that each patient needs to be on the medication that safely works best for him or her:

> That being said, I usually begin with natural desiccated thyroid because it most closely mimics the normal thyroid gland. If this is not what the patient feels best on or has objections (for example, those who keep Kosher, or who are vegetarians—since natural desiccated thyroid is a pork-derived product), I use synthetic T4 and T3 alone or in combination. Often compounded T3 is a useful adjunct to T4 when quick-release [manufactured] T3 is not well tolerated or needs to be dosed multiple times a day. I myself feel best on a combination of natural desiccated thyroid and compounded slow-release T3. Everyone is different, and it often takes some experimentation to find the agent or combination of agents that gives the best result.

ARE YOU AT THE OPTIMAL DOSAGE/ TSH LEVEL FOR YOU?

While the "normal" range for TSH lab tests is established for each lab, where you personally feel best can vary. A study reported in the *Journal of Clinical Endocrinology and Metabolism* found that the mean TSH level for people who don't have a thyroid condition is 1.5. The American Association of Clinical Endocrinologists stated that the normal range for TSH tests is 0.3 to 3.0, despite the fact that many practitioners and labs are still using the outdated 0.5 to 5.0 range, leaving millions of people in the 3.0 to 5.0 range undiagnosed, untreated, and at risk of a host of symptoms.

It's no wonder that if your TSH level is on the higher end of normal for you, you may have symptoms. Check your most recent blood test results and consult with your physician about whether a slight increase in dosage and a reduction in your TSH level would be better for your health.

Ultimately, until you take your thyroid medication for a while, you won't know the TSH level at which you will feel your best. It could be 0.3, 3.0, or somewhere in between. But the idea that people feel their best at different TSH levels has not gained widespread acceptance among many endocrinologists or conventional physicians.

So if you are seeing a doctor who still goes by the old 0.5 to 5.5 range, he or she may treat you but provide you with only enough thyroid hormone to get your TSH level to the higher end of the normal range (that is, to 4.0 to 5.0). The doctor may also tell you that if you don't feel well at the high end of normal, then something else is wrong with you because it's not your thyroid, since it's normal. This is a sign that it's time for another doctor.

DO YOU NEED A SEASONAL ADJUSTMENT IN DOSAGE?

One little-known issue for thyroid patients is the seasonal variation in thyroid function. A number of studies show that TSH naturally rises during colder months and drops to low normal or even hyperthyroid levels in the warmest months. Some doctors adjust for this by prescribing slightly increased dosages during colder months and reducing dosage during warm periods. Most doctors and patients are not aware of this seasonal fluctuation, however, leaving patients suffering with worsening hypothyroidism symptoms during colder months or going through warmer months suffering with hyperthyroidism symptoms due to slight overdosage. This seasonal fluctuation becomes more pronounced in older people, particularly those in cold climates. Twice-yearly tests, at minimum, during winter and summer months can help assess fluctuations and guide any seasonal dosage modifications that are needed.

SHOULD YOU TAKE YOUR THYROID MEDICATION MORE THAN ONCE A DAY?

If you are taking a levothyroxine drug, there is no benefit to splitting your dose and taking it multiple times a day. The drug is dissolved so slowly, and has such a long half-life in your body, that there is no benefit to be had by taking it in staggered doses.

For drugs that contain T3, including Cytomel, Thyrolar, Armour, and the other desiccated thyroid drugs, as well as compounded drugs that contain T3, you may in fact want to stagger your dosage throughout the day, to help maintain a steady level and offer the best possible relief of symptoms. T3 is faster-acting and has a short half-life in the body, and some people report better results when they take their thyroid medications two or three times a day. Some patients take a dose in the morning and at bedtime; others take a morning, lunchtime, and bedtime dose. Time-released compounded drugs eliminate the need for split dosages by gradually releasing T3 throughout the day.

(You should always discuss any change in the way you take your medication with your physician.)

IS YOUR MEDICATION FLUCTUATING IN POTENCY?

If you've had your brand of thyroid medication changed or a generic prescription refilled since your last thyroid test, you may have a change in symptoms and a fluctuation in your thyroid levels. From brand to brand, there is a significant difference in potency, even among pills of the same dosage, so switching from an 88 mcg pill of one brand name levothyroxine to another can actually result in a change in your symptoms.

There is a risk that if you are prescribed generic levothyroxine, each time you get a prescription refill, you may be given a thyroid medication from a different manufacturer. This is the key reason why most practitioners recommend that you not use generic levothyroxine. If you have no choice and must get generic levothyroxine, try to personally work with a pharmacist who will ensure that you get the same product from the same manufacturer.

ARE YOU DELIBERATELY BEING UNDERDOSED?

Some physicians make it a practice to underdose thyroid medication. This means that they will prescribe a patient just enough thyroid medication to get the TSH level into the top end of whichever normal range they use, even though many practitioners recognize that the majority of patients feel best at a level more like the general population's average TSH of 1.0 to 2.0.

The main reason for this policy of underdosing is the fear of osteoporosis, which was discussed earlier in the chapter. Practitioners are mistakenly concerned that maintaining a woman's TSH level at a level of, say, 1.0 to 2.0, rather than above 4.0, is a risk factor for osteoporosis. Meanwhile, if you're being treated but your TSH is still in the high normal range (and I consider that to be 3.0 and above), then you may not feel well.

If your doctor has this philosophy, you may be able to get him or her to work with you on increasing the dosage by agreeing to have periodic bone densitometry testing to assure your doctor that the medication is not having an adverse effect.

ARE YOU TAKING YOUR MEDICATION PROPERLY AND CONSISTENTLY?

There are a number of guidelines on how to properly take thyroid hormone, to ensure that you are absorbing the drug and receiving the maximum possible benefit.

- Don't take thyroid hormone replacement within four hours of taking calcium supplements or drinking calcium-fortified juice. The same rule applies for antacids, such as Tums and Mylanta in liquid or tablet form, which also contain calcium and can delay or reduce the absorption of thyroid hormone.

- Don't take thyroid hormone replacement within four hours of taking any supplements that contain iron.

- Don't take thyroid medication until it's been at least an hour since you've had coffee. The acids in coffee can interfere with thyroid hormone absorption. Try to take thyroid hormone around the same time each day. For best results, maximum absorption, and minimum interference from food, fiber, and supplements, doctors recommend taking it in the morning on an empty stomach, about an hour before eating. Some new studies have shown, however, that the best absorption may be achieved if the medication is taken at bedtime, at least two hours since last eating. Because bowels slow down during the night, the medication makes a slower transit, allowing for maximum absorption. (Note: Some thyroid patients find that taking T3 medication at night may disrupt sleep. Others find that a small dose of T3 at bedtime helps improve sleep quality.)

- If you need to take thyroid hormone with food, be consistent and *always* take it with food. Don't switch between taking it with and without food, because switching will cause erratic absorption, and it will be harder to regulate your TSH levels.

-- If you start or stop a high-fiber diet while you are on thyroid hormone, have your thyroid function retested around six to eight weeks after your dietary change. High-fiber diets can change the speed of thyroid drug absorption, and you may require a dosage adjustment. You should also be consistent about your daily fiber intake. Don't take 10 grams one day, 30 grams the next day, and so on, or you're risking erratic absorption.

-- If you are on the Levoxyl brand of levothyroxine, take the drug with enough water and swallow the pill quickly. The pill dissolves rapidly, so if it dissolves completely in your mouth, you risk not absorbing all of the active ingredients.

Any time you have a dramatic dietary change, for example, starting or stopping a high-fiber diet or starting or no longer taking your thyroid medication with food, get your thyroid levels retested about six to eight weeks later, to ensure you're receiving the proper amount of thyroid hormone.

ARE OTHER MEDICATIONS INTERFERING WITH OR INTERACTING WITH YOUR THYROID MEDICATION?

Use of tricyclic antidepressants such as doxepin, amitriptyline, desipramine, and imipramine (brand names include Adapin, Elavil, Norpramin, and Tofranil) at the same time as thyroid hormone may increase the effects of both drugs and may accelerate the effects of the antidepressant. Be sure your doctor knows you are on one before prescribing the other.

Also, researchers have found that taking thyroid hormone replacement while taking the popular antidepressant sertraline (brand name Zoloft) can cause a decrease in the effectiveness of the thyroid hormone replacement. This same effect has been seen in patients receiving other selective serotonin reuptake inhibitors such as paroxetine (brand name Paxil) and fluoxetine (brand name Prozac).

If you are taking an antidepressant and your doctor prescribes thyroid medication (or vice versa), be sure to get your thyroid retested six to eight weeks after starting the new medication to evaluate any possible interactions.

A number of other drugs may interact with thyroid hormone or affect thyroid function:

- **Insulin:** thyroid hormone can reduce the effectiveness of insulin and similar drugs for diabetes. Be sure your doctor knows you are on one before prescribing the other.

- **Cholesterol-lowering drugs cholestyramine and colestipol:** these drugs (brand names include Colestrol, Questran, and Colestid) bind thyroid hormone. A minimum of four to five hours should elapse between taking these drugs and thyroid hormone.

- **Anticoagulants ("blood thinners"):** anticoagulant drugs like warfarin (brand name Coumadin) and heparin can sometimes become stronger in the system when thyroid hormone is added to the mix. Mention it to your doctor if you are on one or the other.

- **Corticosteroids/adrenocorticosteroids:** brands include Cortisone, Cortistab, and Cortone. These drugs suppress TSH and can block conversion of T4 to T3 in some people.

- **Amiodarone hydrochloride (HCL):** the heart drug amiodarone HCL (brand name Cordarone) can cause hypothyroidism or hyperthyroidism and interfere with T4 metabolism. People taking Cordarone should be monitored periodically for thyroid changes.

- **Ketamine:** some patients taking ketamine, a drug used as an anesthetic (and illegally as a recreational hallucinogen known as "K" or "Special K"), experience elevated blood pressure and a racing heart when taking levothyroxine sodium and ketamine at the same time.

- **Maprotiline:** this antidepressant can increase the risk of cardiac arrhythmias when taken with thyroid hormone products.

- **Theophylline:** this drug for asthma and respiratory diseases may not clear out of the body as quickly when someone is hypothyroid, but it usually clears normally when TSH is in the normal range.

- **Lithium:** used to treat bipolar disease and some forms of depression, lithium is known to actually create hypothyroidism by blocking secretion of T4 and T3. People taking lithium should be monitored periodically for thyroid changes.

- **Phenytoin:** this anticonvulsant, a brand of which is Dilantin, may accelerate levothyroxine metabolism, and tests may show decreased total T4 levels.

- **Carbamazepine:** this anticonvulsant pain medicine, a brand of which is Tegretol, may accelerate levothyroxine metabolism, and tests may show decreased total T4 levels.

- **Rifampin:** this antituberculosis agent may accelerate levothyroxine metabolism, and tests may show decreased total T4 levels.

ARE YOU FORGETTING TO TAKE YOUR MEDICATION?

Surprisingly, one of the key reasons patients don't feel well on thyroid treatment is that they are failing to take their medications regularly, as prescribed. When you are on thyroid hormone replacement, it's critical that you take your medication every day as prescribed. Even a day or two's failure to take thyroid medication can throw off your treatment regimen and have a dramatic effect on your overall health. Here are some tips on how to remember to take your medication.

– Write it in your datebook in a bright color that is hard to miss.

– If you use a computer, cell phone, or personal digital assistant

(PDA) like a Palm Pilot or BlackBerry, consider adding a reminder in the scheduling program. Some programs allow you to set a regular daily "appointment" at a particular time. Some even have an alarm function you can set to remind you.

— Put a message on your computer's screen saver.

— Keep your thyroid drug pill container near your alarm clock, so you can remember to take your medicine first thing in the morning. (But be careful to keep your medications away from children.)

— Link taking your medicine with key daily events, such as brushing your teeth in the morning.

— Put a note wherever you'll notice it every day—on the refrigerator, coffee maker, toothbrush holder, or bathroom vanity mirror.

— Take your medicine the same time every day, so it becomes a habit.

— Hire a calling service to give you a daily "wakeup" call to remind you to take your pill. If you have a home voicemail answering system such as AnswerCall, you can program a daily reminder call at the same time each day. You can even sign up online for free services like Wakerupper.com, which will make free reminder calls to you.

— Use a pill sorter, or a device known as a dosette, which has compartments for different days or even different times of the day.

— Get a special device to remind you to take your pill. You can get medication computers, vibrating watches, automatic dispensers, beepers, and other alarms that can help keep you on schedule.

– Enlist the aid of a family member or friend. Sometimes, just a few weeks of friendly reminders can help you get into the habit of taking your medicine at the right time every day.

Nutrition and Supplements for Thyroid Function

You'll want to make sure that you are getting proper nutritional supplements to help support your thyroid.

MULTIVITAMINS

A high-potency multivitamin is essential for thyroid patients. Look for one that has high amounts of B vitamins, vitamin C, vitamin E, and a good range of minerals. One that I particularly like is Dr. Jacob Teitelbaum's formulation known as Daily Energy Enfusion. Dr. Teitelbaum's multivitamin formula does contain some iodine, however, so you may want to slightly reduce your daily dosage if you are iodine sensitive. It comes as a flavorful powdered drink along with one vitamin B capsule, and is the equivalent of more than thirty vitamins and supplement pills that would need to be taken each day. Daily Energy Enfusion does not include iron or calcium, so it can be taken at the same time as thyroid hormone.

Specifically, you want to make sure you are getting

- Vitamin A: a deficiency in vitamin A may limit the ability to produce thyroid hormone.
- Vitamin B_2 (riboflavin): a shortage of vitamin B_2 can depress endocrine function, especially the thyroid and adrenals.
- Vitamin B_3 (niacin): vitamin B_3 helps keep cells working by aiding in respiration and delivery of energy to cells.
- Vitamin B_6 (pyridoxine): vitamin B_6 helps the body convert iodine to thyroid hormone.
- Vitamin B_{12} (cyanocobalamin, methylcobalamin): hypothyroidism causes the body to be less able to absorb sufficient B_{12} from diet alone. Some experts recommend patients with hypothyroidism

get 1,000 to 5,000 mg (milligrams) of vitamin B_{12} daily, even via injection. Sublingual (under the tongue) B_{12} is a more effective form of delivery than other B_{12} supplements.

- **Vitamin E**: vitamin E is an essential antioxidant and can help with immune function.

VITAMIN C

Many experts recommend that in addition to your multivitamin, you take 2,000 to 3,000 mg of vitamin C each day. You can use capsules or powdered forms of vitamin C.

One particular favorite of mine is Emergen-C drink mix. It's very low in calories and sugar but very flavorful (I particularly like the raspberry, cranberry, and tangerine flavors.) Each envelope makes one drink, and the drink has a bit of fizz to it, so it functions like a soda. But it's packed with 1,000 mg (1 gram) of vitamin C, as well as B_6, B_{12}, potassium, and a variety of other useful vitamins.

VITAMIN D

Vitamin D functions as a hormone and is necessary for the pituitary gland to produce thyroid hormone; it may also play a role in T3 binding to its receptor. It enables the deiodinase enzyme to convert T4 (inactive thyroid hormone) to T3 (the active type). It is also thought that vitamin D is necessary for health immune system functioning.

PROBIOTICS

Probiotics are supplements that contain live bacteria—the "good" bacteria found in fermented foods such as miso and in dairy products such as yogurt and some cheeses. These bacteria are needed in sufficient quantities in the intestinal system. One probiotic bacterium is *Acidophilus*, the live culture found in yogurt.

The probiotic bacteria known as *Bifidobacterium lactis* HN019 reportedly boosts the activity of various disease-killing immune system cells in healthy adults. Probiotics aid proper digestive functioning, which enhances the immune system. They also kill off harmful bacteria, having an antibiotic effect by fighting off various types of infection. You can eat yogurt, but the concentration of live cultures in yogurt is not high enough to get a substantial enough effect, so a probiotic supplement is your best option. Some probiotic supplements can be expensive and require refrigeration, but I recommend a patented formula from Enzymatic Therapies called Acidophilus Pearls. This tiny pearl-shaped supplement contains a guaranteed level of live bacteria in the millions, is very inexpensive, and requires no refrigeration.

ZINC

Zinc is needed by the thyroid for both hormone production and T4-to-T3 conversion. It is also necessary for proper hypothalamic functioning, an essential part of thyroid function. Zinc, along with selenium, can help prevent the decline of T3, which can occur on a low-calorie diet.

SELENIUM

Perhaps the most important mineral for thyroid function is selenium. Selenium activates hepatic type I iodothyronine deiodinase, which is responsible for controlling thyroid function by the conversion of T4 to T3. This enzyme is a selenoprotein that is sensitive to selenium deficiency. Stress and injury appear to make the body particularly selenium-deficient. After severe injury, the conversion of T4 to T3 is decreased, leading to low T3 syndrome. One study found that selenium levels are low after trauma, which correlates to low T3 levels, along with a decrease in the T4-to-T3 conversion.

Some researchers and practitioners are beginning to believe that selenium deficiency alone can trigger autoimmune thyroid disease in some people. One study published in 2002 showed that in areas with severe selenium deficiency, there is a higher incidence of autoimmune thyroiditis. In the study, patients with thyroid antibodies received 200 mcg of selenium supplementation over three months. At the end of the test period, antibody levels had decreased by as much as 40 to 63 percent; a small percentage of patients in the selenium-treated group had antibody levels that completely returned to normal. The researchers concluded that selenium supplementation may reduce inflammation in patients with autoimmune thyroiditis.

A 1997 study found that high intake of iodine—when selenium is deficient—could trigger thyroid damage. But sufficient intake of selenium appeared to offset the dangers of high iodine intake.

Experts recommend 200 mcg of selenium a day but caution that selenium is one of those supplements where more is *not* better. Overdosage on selenium can be harmful, so keep your intake to 200 to 400 mcg, maximum.

MAGNESIUM

Magnesium is an essential mineral that is often deficient in thyroid patients. It helps maintain normal muscle and nerve function, keeps heart rhythm steady, and strengthens bones. It is also involved in energy metabolism. If you aren't getting enough magnesium, you may have more muscle cramps and pain than usual, as well as tingling, numbness, and abnormal heart rhythms—all symptoms that are also more common in thyroid patients.

TYROSINE

Tyrosine is considered the precursor to T4 thyroid hormone. The thyroid takes in iodine and combines that iodine with the amino acid tyrosine, converting the iodine/tyrosine combination into T3 and T4. So a deficiency in tyrosine means a basic building block of good thyroid function is missing.

GUGGUL

Z-guggulsterone (known as guggul), a component derived from the plant *Commiphora mukul*, has been used in Ayurvedic medicine as an anti-inflammatory, antiobesity, thyroid-stimulating, and cholesterol-lowering agent. Guggul is considered particularly important for prevention of a sluggish metabolism, and may increase the thyroid's ability take up the enzymes it needs for effective hormone conversion and also increase the oxygen uptake in muscles. Some people find that guggul is overstimulating, so you need to be careful using this supplement.

ASHWAGANDHA

Ashwagandha (*Withania somnifera*), also known as Indian ginseng and winter cherry, is an adaptogenic herb traditionally used to improve fertility, increase sex drive, and enhance the immune system. Some studies have shown that ashwagandha stimulates thyroid activity and may help fight fatigue in thyroid patients.

ESSENTIAL FATTY ACIDS

Essential fatty acids are critical for thyroid patients. Many practitioners recommend them to reduce inflammation—particularly important in autoimmune-triggered hypothyroidism. Essential fatty acids cannot be produced in the body, so you must get them through diet or supplements. The key essential fatty acids include

- Omega-3/alpha-linolenic acid (ALA), eicosapentaenoic acid (EPA), docosahexaenoic acid (DHA): found in fresh fish from cold, deep waters (for example, mackerel, tuna, herring, flounder, sardines, salmon, rainbow trout, and bass), linseed oil, flaxseeds and flaxseed oil, black currant and pumpkin seeds, cod liver oil, shrimp, oysters, leafy greens, soybeans, walnuts, wheat germ, fresh sea vegetables, and fish oil. Usually, your body can convert ALA into EPA, then into DHA.
- Omega-6/linoleic acid/gamma linolenic acid (GLA): found in breast milk; sesame, safflower, cotton, and sunflower seeds and oil; corn and corn oil; soybeans; raw nuts; legumes; leafy greens; black currant seeds; evening primrose oil (EPO), borage oil; spirulina; and lecithin. Linoleic acid in omega-6 can be converted into GLA.

Besides adding more of the foods that contain these essential fatty acids to your diet, you can add the following:

- **Omega-3/fish oil supplements:** go for a decent tasting oil or a "burpless" capsule (Enzymatic Therapies' Eskimo Oil is my favorite).
- **Omega-3/flaxseeds and flaxseed oil:** you can add flaxseed to your meals, either in the oil form or as capsules. Some people like to make salad dressings with the oil or add it to soups. Taking flaxseed oil with each meal helps slow down digestion and modulate blood sugar fluctuations (which helps with insulin levels).
- **Omega-6/evening primrose oil, borage oil:** these are usually taken as supplements. They are thought to help activate brown fat (a type of fat that generates body heat and raises metabolism) and boost metabolic efficiency. Some practitioners and patients find omega-6 oils to be particularly helpful with hair- and skin-related symptoms of hypothyroidism.

IODINE

Iodine supplementation is a controversial topic for thyroid patients. On the one hand, too little iodine can cause a variety of thyroid problems. On the other hand, too much iodine can trigger or worsen thyroid problems.

The key is knowing if you need iodine supplementation, and if so, how best to take it.

Holistic and nutritional practitioners sometimes assume that every thyroid patient needs iodine or an iodine-containing herb like bladderwrack (*Fucus vesiculosus*), seaweed, or kelp. But there is controversy over the amount of iodine deficiency in the United States. Statistics show that one-fourth to one-third of Americans may have some degree of iodine deficiency. Some practitioners, however, like Michigan's Dr. David Brownstein, one of the pioneers in iodine testing and therapy, say that the vast majority of thyroid patients test positive for iodine deficiency. According to Dr. Brownstein, patients who show suboptimal iodine levels and receive iodine supplementation treatment usually find that their symptoms improve.

Should you take iodine? Answering that question requires that you be tested and, if you are deficient, carefully trying iodine supplementation under the direction of a practitioner.

The best tool for evaluating iodine levels is the urinary iodine clearance test. Dr. Brownstein uses Hakala Research, a laboratory that has pioneered the urinary iodine clearance testing process. For those patients who are iodine deficient, Dr. Brownstein has them follow a protocol for iodine supplementation that uses a specialized combination and dosage of iodine and iodide, designed for best absorption of the nutrient. The combination is found in a pill format, known as Iodoral, and in a liquid called Lugol's solution.

Dr. Brownstein has outlined an entire program for iodine testing and supplementation in his book *Iodine: Why You Need It, Why You Can't Live without It* and I highly recommend that anyone interested in iodine testing and supplementation read this book to learn how to get properly tested and safely supplement with iodine.

Some Cautions

Ensuring that you are getting proper thyroid treatment also means that you must keep certain cautions in mind.

WATCH GOITROGENS

Goitrogens are chemicals in certain products and foods that promote formation of goiters. They can act like antithyroid drugs in slowing down the thyroid and causing hypothyroidism. Specifically, goitrogens inhibit the body's ability to use iodine, block the process by which iodine becomes the thyroid hormones T4 and T3, inhibit the actual secretion of thyroid hormone, and disrupt the peripheral conversion of T4 to T3 in the thyroid gland.

If you don't have a thyroid due to surgery or RAI treatment, you don't have to be particularly concerned about goitrogens. If you still have an even partially functional thyroid, however, you need to be more concerned and careful not to eat goitrogens uncooked in large quantities. The enzymes involved in the formation of goitrogenic materials in plants can be partially destroyed by cooking. Eating moderate amounts of goitrogenic foods, raw or cooked, is probably not a problem for most people.

A list of goitrogenic foods is featured in Chapter 2.

REDUCE TOXIC EXPOSURES

Reduce exposure to fluoride by drinking bottled water that is not fluoridated. Use a fluoride-free toothpaste, and do not get dental fluoride treatments. These have not been clearly demonstrated to be helpful at reducing or preventing cavities in adults.

There's not much you can do to avoid eating perchlorate-contaminated foods, except to grow your own produce and use water that you've had tested for perchlorate contamination. If you drink well water, you should also have that water tested, and if you live in an area near a current or former facility for rockets, explosives, or fireworks production, consider having your water independently tested. Most importantly, become aware of the issues, and monitor the status of perchlorate legislation, by monitoring the comprehensive site www.perchlorate.org.

Regarding mercury, some patients have reported that their thyroid problems and other symptoms were greatly relieved with supplements to help chelate the mercury, and by removing mercury fillings in their teeth. A holistic physician can guide you in evaluating your mercury levels and in deciding what to do in response to elevated levels.

TREAT INFECTIONS

Infection is thought to trigger some thyroid problems. The food-borne bacteria *Yersinia enterocolitica*, for example, has been associated with production and elevated levels of thyroid antibodies, a sign of autoimmune thyroid disease.

A Genova Diagnostics (formerly Great Smokies) laboratory analysis can help detect intestinal bacterial overgrowth that may be contributing to underlying immune system problems and fueling the thyroid condition. These are typically treated with antibiotics, or, if you are working with a more holistic practitioner, diet, nutritional supplements, and herbs that function in an antibiotic-like capacity.

BE CAREFUL OF SOY, ISOFLAVONES, AND PHYTOESTROGENS

Experts can't seem to agree on the subject, and there is much debate regarding the pros and cons of soy. But there is increasing agreement that overconsumption of isoflavone-intensive soy products may trigger or aggravate a thyroid condition. I discuss soy at greater length in Chapter 6, but be aware that overconsumption of isoflavone-intensive soy products (most often this is due to the use or overuse of soy supplements, protein powders, and other processed soy products) may trigger hypothyroidism or worsen an existing thyroid condition. If you are going to use soy, better to use fermented forms of soy foods, like tempeh, tofu, and miso, and only occasionally. A daily diet of soy milk, soy burgers, edamame, soy shakes, and soy foods at every meal elevates soy from mild phytoestrogen to potent hormone that has the ability to harm your hormonal health.

An Important Note for Women Taking Estrogen and Thyroid Hormone Replacement Medication

If you are taking thyroid medication, and you start taking any estrogen medication—that includes birth control pills and all forms of estrogen therapy—you may need to adjust your thyroid dosage as a result of the estrogen.

Estrogen can block thyroid receptors, making your thyroid medication less effective, which may result in the need for an increased dosage.

The drop in estrogen after surgical or natural menopause can also destabilize thyroid dosage requirements. Amanda was on thyroid medication for hypothyroidism when she had a total hysterectomy at age forty-eight. Says Amanda:

Prior to my surgery, I asked my gynecologist if I would have to have my thyroid medication adjusted after surgery, because I know that all of our hormones are well synchronized, and if all of a sudden there is a sudden drop in estrogen (surgical menopause), surely there would be other changes. She assured me that there was no connection and I needn't worry! Needless to say, there is a connection, and I had terrible hormonal problems for a year and many medication adjustments. My thyroid medication had to be increased significantly.

If you add any estrogen medication, be sure to have your thyroid function thoroughly reevaluated (that means not just TSH, but also free T4 and free T3) to see if you require a dosage adjustment.

chapter 5

Diagnosing and Treating

PERIMENOPAUSE/ MENOPAUSE

The best mind-altering drug is truth.

—*Lily Tomlin*

The key diagnosis of perimenopause or menopause is done by

- Irregularity or absence of menstrual periods
- Characteristic symptoms, including hot flashes and night sweats

The following section looks at some of the more specific evaluations that can be done to help confirm that perimenopause is under way or that menopause has taken place.

Self-Checks

MENSTRUAL/SYMPTOM TRACKING

In terms of self-checks, one of the main ways you can evaluate perimenopause is to keep a menstrual chart and symptoms diary.

Monthly tracking of the menstrual cycle and symptoms can help to identify perimenopausal patterns (more or less frequent periods and other changes that are common in perimenopause.)

In addition to tracking the start and stop dates of menstruation, you should keep track of menstrual characteristics, such as heaviness/lightness of flow, presence of clots, menstrual color (brown or red), and spotting. Also keep track of symptoms such as cramps, bloating, headache/migraine, hot flashes, night sweats, insomnia, cravings, excessive fatigue, vaginal discharge, vaginal odor, and vaginal itching.

You may also want to note any of the following symptoms:

- Discharge from breasts
- Facial hair
- Changes in your weight

You can use your BlackBerry or Palm Pilot, computer calendar, or organizer for tracking. You will also find printable tracking charts for your use online at the book's Web site at www.menopausethyroid .com.

MENOPAUSE TEST KIT

The Early Detect Menopause Home Test Kit, available at drugstores, is a simple urine test to determine if menopause has begun. The kit measures the amount of follicle-stimulating hormone (FSH) in your urine.

FSH is not considered a conclusive test to diagnose menopause, but if high FSH levels are identified on a number of occasions over a several-month period, it can help to support suspicion of perimenopause or menopause. Taking hormones, including birth control, can make this test inaccurate and inconclusive.

THE CLINICAL PERIMENOPAUSE/MENOPAUSE EXAMINATION

Ideally, your doctor should perform a physical examination, including a pelvic exam, to check you for conditions that may contribute to menstrual irregularities or symptoms. If you are pre- or perimenopausal, a Pap smear and pregnancy test are also frequently done. The pelvic exam may reveal some of the following characteristic changes that can confirm perimenopause or menopause.

- Changes to color and appearance of the epithelial layer of the vagina
- Smoothing of vaginal wall
- Shrinking of uterus
- Reduction in the size of the ovary
- Inability to palpate ovary
- Prolapse of reproductive or urinary tract organs

A thorough physician will attempt to rule out gynecological conditions that can cause menstrual irregularities and problems, including

- Vaginal infection
- Tumors, polyps, fibroids, and cysts of the vagina, cervix, uterus, ovaries, or fallopian tubes
- Cervical disorders
- Cancer of the uterus, cervix, vagina, vulva, or bladder
- Sexually transmitted diseases, for example, chlamydia, gonorrhea, and human papillomavirus (HPV)/genital warts
- Pregnancy (normal or ectopic)
- Endometriosis, a condition in which the tissue that normally lines the uterus grows outside the uterus
- Pelvic inflammatory disease (PID), a sexually transmitted infection
- Scarring or adhesions from previous surgeries

- Turner's syndrome, a birth defect related to the reproductive system
- Inflammatory bowel disease (IBD)
- Pituitary growth or tumor

Urinalysis is also done, and perimenopausal and menopausal women frequently show a decrease in the pH of urine.

Perimenopause/Menopause Blood Tests

There is no definitive or conclusive blood test for perimenopause or menopause. All we can do is monitor certain hormones, along with symptoms and menstrual history, to get a sense of what is going on.

The main blood tests that are conventionally used to evaluate the perimenopausal and menopausal hormone status are FSH, LH, and estradiol (E2) levels.

Integrative practitioners and women's hormone experts tend to also test the other hormones in the pathway, including progesterone, testosterone, and DHEA-sulfate (DHEA-S).

FOLLICLE-STIMULATING HORMONE

The FSH blood test measures the level of follicle-stimulating hormone. This test is considered inconclusive during perimenopause because the levels can fluctuate dramatically from month to month, and blood FSH levels don't correlate particularly with perimenopausal symptoms such as hot flashes.

Also, keep in mind, one "postmenopausal" FSH level does not mean that the period will not return, or that a woman is not still having a menstrual cycle (even if it's erratic), or that a woman cannot still become pregnant.

When the FSH test consistently shows levels above ovulation range, along with cessation of menstrual periods, this is considered to be confirmation that menopause has taken place. But it's really verifying what you know after the fact.

Generally, however, while levels can fluctuate during a woman's cycle,

- FSH levels consistently above 15 to 25 IU/L may be perimenopausal
- FSH levels consistently above 30 to 50 IU/L are considered menopausal

LUTEINIZING HORMONE

Luteinizing hormone, the hormone that surges right before ovulation (and that is measured by ovulation detector kits), can rise to levels as high as 25 to 60 milli International Units per milliliter (mIU/mL) during perimenopause. Levels consistently above 40 are considered menopausal, however.

ESTROGEN

Estradiol (E2) is a key form of estrogen, and the one whose fluctuation typically causes the most perimenopausal/menopausal symptoms. Some integrative or hormone-oriented practitioners also test estrone (E1) and estriol (E3), the other types of estrogen.

Estrogen levels, however, don't correlate especially well with symptoms. Some women have high levels but are symptomatic because their levels have dropped from even higher levels. Other women can have very low estrogen levels and not suffer from typical menopause symptoms.

For the purposes of confirmation, estradiol levels consistently below 20 to 30 picograms per milliliter (pg/mL) may be associated with perimenopause or menopause.

OTHER HORMONES

Normal ranges of other hormones depend on the lab where the tests are being done and how the hormone levels are measured. Measuring progesterone, testosterone, and DHEA doesn't really help diagnose perimenopause or menopause, but it can be done to help assess deficiencies that might be addressed through hormone support. For DHEA, the most accurate test is the DHEA-S.

ORDERING YOUR OWN TESTS

You have several options for hormonal testing that do not require a doctor's lab orders or, in one case, even a venous (from a vein) blood draw.

You can get ZRT Labs' blood spot testing, which you can do at home with blood you get from a nearly painless finger prick. ZRT tests for a number of hormones and values, including

- Estradiol
- Progesterone
- Luteinizing hormone
- Follicle-stimulating hormone
- Testosterone
- DHEA-S

Individual and combination test kits are offered by ZRT. (ZRT also has blood spot testing for various thyroid values and saliva cortisol, among other tests.) No doctor's prescription is needed. (Due to state regulations, ZRT can provide testing in California and New York only with a doctor's prescription.)

MyMedLab is a direct-to-consumer service that allows you to request any blood test in a long list of common tests; you do not need a lab slip to order the tests. You then go to a local collection site for LabCorp, the national testing laboratory used by many doctors, to have the blood drawn (or to provide the urine sample or other testing sample). You pay a much lower discounted rate for tests, due to MyMedLab's negotiated prices, and the results of the tests are given to you directly, including in a secure online chart that tracks results over time.

MyMedLab offers hundreds of different tests, but the relevant reproductive hormone tests available are

- Estradiol (E2)
- Estrone (E1)
- Estriol (E3)
- Progesterone
- Luteinizing hormone
- Follicle-stimulating hormone
- Testosterone
- DHEA-S

MyMedLab has its own doctors who sign off on lab requests. Due to state regulations, MyMedLab is unable to process direct-to-consumer testing in New York, New Jersey, and Rhode Island.

Information on ZRT and MyMedLab is featured in Appendix A and at the book's Web site, www.menopausethyroid.com.

Imaging and Diagnostic Tests

If symptoms are especially significant, or if menstrual irregularities are severe (that is, you experience continuous menstrual bleeding), some physicians may require additional tests and diagnostic procedures to look for cysts, fibroids, and tumors or to obtain samples for evaluation. Tests include computed tomography (CT) scan ("cat" scan), magnetic resonance imaging (MRI), ultrasound, endometrial biopsy, laparoscopy and hysteroscopy, and dilation and curettage (known as D&C).

Diagnosing Perimenopause/Menopause

Evaluation of menstrual problems requires that your doctor take a complete medical history. This should include information regarding your puberty, first menstrual period, menstrual cycle, symptoms, and the menstrual, fertility, and menopausal patterns of your mother, grandmothers, and any sisters.

Based on your personal and family history, symptoms, menstrual tracking, clinical examination, and, potentially, blood tests, a doctor can make a presumptive diagnosis of perimenopause or menopause. (Keep in mind that, except in the case of surgical removal of the female reproductive organs, a firm diagnosis of menopause is mostly retrospective, in that the periods have to have stopped for a full year.)

The Precursor Hormones

PREGNENOLONE

For supplementation, bioidentical pregnenolone (pregnenolone that is chemically identical to the body's own pregnenolone) is available in higher-potency prescription forms from compounding pharmacies, typically in capsules, or in transdermal forms like gels and creams.

Pregnenolone is also available over the counter in capsules and tablets, and as an ingredient in over-the-counter transdermal creams.

Regarding the "parent hormone" pregnenolone, some practitioners claim that it is safe at any dose; others are concerned about long-term high-dose use. The truth is, there really aren't any studies that look at the long-term effects of pregnenolone, and you'll want to supplement it only with the guidance of your practitioner. Many holistic practitioners suggest that supplementation of pregnenolone for women not exceed 5 to 10 mg a day.

Pregnenolone can have some side effects, even at low doses, including

- Irregular heart rhythms and palpitations
- Acne
- Irritability, anxiety
- Hair loss
- Insomnia
- Headaches

DEHYDROEPIANDROSTERONE (DHEA)

When you are deficient in DHEA, bioidentical DHEA is available in higher-potency prescription forms from compounding pharmacies, in capsule, or in transdermal forms like gels and creams.

DHEA also became available to the public without a prescription after the 1994 passage of the U.S. Dietary Supplement Health and Education Act. It is available in capsule and tablet form and is also an ingredient in over-the-counter transdermal creams.

Because over-the-counter DHEA supplements and creams are unregulated, you can't be assured that they contain the stated amount of DHEA, if any. Several practitioners who regularly recommend over-the-counter DHEA, however, have suggested the Youthful You DHEA formulation by Enzymatic Therapies, as a high-quality, pharmaceutical-grade DHEA.

Long-term use of DHEA hasn't been studied. As with pregnenolone, there are varying claims about the safety of different dosages and long-term use but few studies that look at the long-term use or impact on other hormones.

DHEA can have some side effects, even at doses as low as 5 to 10 mg a day, including

- Irregular heart rhythms and palpitations
- Acne
- Irritability, anxiety
- Hair loss
- Insomnia
- Headaches
- Increased body odor
- Menstrual irregularities

Because DHEA converts to testosterone, taking excessive levels of DHEA is associated with symptoms of excess testosterone in women, which include growth of facial hair and deepening of the voice.

Even though DHEA is available over the counter, most experts I spoke with agreed that you should not self-treat with DHEA. Instead, be sure to get blood work to evaluate DHEA-S levels. If your levels are borderline or low, you may then want to try low-dose DHEA supplementation with a high-quality DHEA. Some practitioners recommend that most women not exceed 5 mg a day of DHEA.

According to Dr. Uzzi Reiss, Beverly Hills, California, gynecologist and author of *The Natural Superwoman*, most women can take from 5 to 15 mg of DHEA without side effects. Says Dr. Reiss:

> Take DHEA during the morning (start with 5 mg). If you have side effects: chin hair growth, head hair loss, acne skin breakouts, or oily skin, then lower the dosage. If you can, increase the dosage, but don't exceed 15 mg. If you experience any edginess or agitation, this is also a symptom of too much, so drop back down.

PROGESTERONE

Progesterone drugs—known as progestogens—include synthetic progesterone analogues (called progestins) and a natural, bioidentical progesterone.

For women who still have a uterus and are taking any estrogen treatment, progestogens help prevent endometrial hyperplasia (overgrowth of the uterine lining), a condition that can increase the risk of endometrial and uterine cancer.

The most commonly prescribed form of progestogen therapy is the progestin known as medroxyprogesterone. The brand name of the oral form is Provera, and it is also available in a generic form.

Other oral progestins are

- Micronor and Nor-QD and generic norethindrone
- Aygestin and generic norethindrone acetate
- Ovrette and generic norgestrel
- Megace and generic megestrol acetate

Mirena is an intrauterine device (IUD) that delivers levonorgestrel, a synthesized progestin.

Progestin-only contraceptive pills ("mini-pills") are also available, including Micronor, Nora-BE, and Nor-QD. Norplant is a high-dose contraceptive progestin implant; Depo-Provera is a high-dose contraceptive delivered by injection.

The other key type of progestogen therapy is bioidentical progesterone, which is available in several manufactured forms:

- Prometrium, an oral micronized progesterone capsule, suspended in peanut oil
- Prochieve and Crinone, vaginal progesterone gels

Compounding pharmacies offer a variety of forms and strengths of bioidentical progesterone, including

- Oral capsules
- Transdermal creams, to be rubbed into the skin
- Vaginal creams
- Vaginal suppositories
- Sublingual pills or drops, to dissolve under the tongue
- Troches (lozenges that dissolve between the cheek and gum)
- Implantable pellets

With oral micronized progesterone, keep in mind that higher doses may be necessary to help regulate the menstrual cycle, or to cause bleeding. For example, doses above 200 mg are generally thought to produce a more predictable cycle, but doses as high as 300 to 400 mg may be needed to cause withdrawal bleeding (which is sometimes called for if you are on estrogen).

Progesterone cream in a lower strength is also sold over the counter, without a prescription. There are dozens of progesterone creams on the market, but most practitioners who recommend over-the-counter progesterone cream to their patients typically suggest they use a reputable, quality-controlled brand, ProGest Cream, which is manufactured by Emerita. The ConsumerLab Web site has reviewed several brands of progesterone, including Balance Progesterone Naturally cream and Kevala's PureGest, and verified that they contain the stated level of hormone.

For over-the-counter progesterone creams, practitioners typically recommend that you use ¼ to ½ teaspoon of progesterone cream (with a goal of providing 20 to 40 mg of progesterone), starting anywhere from the eighth day of the cycle. (Day 1 is the first day of menstruation.) You continue to apply the cream until day 26 of the cycle, then stop. If you have a period, start again on day 8. If you don't have a period, wait for nine days, and start again, counting it as day 1.

(Note: Some practitioners have you add another ¼ teaspoon from day 14 through day 26 of the cycle to increase progesterone levels.)

For women who take progesterone, because it can have a sedative effect, most practitioners recommend that you take or use it thirty minutes to an hour before bedtime. (If you are new to progesterone, you may want to start taking it on a day when you don't have a grueling schedule or an early start the next day, so that you can see whether it makes you especially tired.)

From a conventional perspective, the only reason for progestogen therapy is to "oppose" estrogen. This means, if you are taking estrogen and you still have a uterus, you need to take a progestogen to help reduce the endometrial thickening—and its risk of cancer— that is associated with taking estrogen.

There are downsides to taking synthetic progestin drugs. They appear to be associated with an increased risk of breast cancer. There are a number of other side effects that are reportedly linked to progestins, including

- Menstrual irregularities, breakthrough bleeding
- Weight gain
- Bloating
- Breast tenderness

- Dizziness
- Disrupted sleep
- Morning drowsiness
- Fatigue
- Muscle/joint pain
- Acne
- Migraines
- Depression
- Mood swings
- Irritability
- Increased insulin resistance
- Bone loss

It's controversial, but some practitioners believe that medroxy-progesterone acetate in particular, the ingredient in Prempro, may actually cause vascular toxicity, including blood vessel damage, tendency to form blood clots, and inflammation.

On the other hand, proponents of natural/bioidentical progesterone claim that most of the significant risks of the progestins are not seen with progesterone. They also believe that progesterone has a number of positive side effects and functions that are beneficial for women.

Dr. Uzzi Reiss is a practitioner who believes that natural progesterone, in contrast to progestins, actually has positive effects and protects against breast cancer, does not affect insulin resistance, helps to build bone, and promotes better sleep.

In addition to counteracting the endometrial buildup that can result from taking any form of estrogen, proponents claim that progesterone can counteract the clotting effects of estrogen, which helps mitigate the stroke and heart risk of estrogen treatment and potentially even helps prevent heart disease.

Proponents also claim that progesterone helps the body better use thyroid hormone. Some proponents feel that bioidentical progesterone alone can relieve menopausal symptoms, especially in women who are suffering from estrogen dominance in menopause, where symptoms may be due to low progesterone rather than estrogen deficiency.

The positive claims about progesterone are a point of controversy, because there simply hasn't been substantial research that proves or disproves these claims. But proponents claim that because the bioidentical form is chemically the same as human progesterone, in balanced and reasonable doses, the supplemental progesterone is no more risky than the body's own hormones.

Some issues remain, however:

– Prometrium, the oral micronized progesterone tablet, is manufactured using peanut oil, so anyone with a peanut allergy can't use it. (Oral micronized progesterone can be compounded in another oil, however, for oral use.)

– Some women react to progesterone, experiencing dizziness or morning drowsiness. For some women, this means that the dose is too high and should be reduced.

– Natural progesterone taken orally is easily degraded by the liver. Very high doses need to be taken in order for it to reach the tissues, and this can put stress on the liver. Some doctors believe that for this reason, transdermal forms of progesterone, such as suppositories, gels, and creams, are preferable.

– There is no evidence that nonprescription/over-the-counter progesterone cream can oppose the negative effects estrogen has on the endometrium, so nonprescription creams are not recommended for use in combination estrogen/progesterone therapies.

TESTOSTERONE

From a conventional standpoint, the only indication for testosterone therapy is to treat decreased sexual desire in women, primarily after menopause. Antiaging practitioners believe that testosterone supplementation can help with energy and muscle building in women.

When supplemental testosterone is needed for a woman, it can be prescribed in several conventional forms:

- Gel form: Androgel, Testim
- Pellet and intramuscular formulations

Oral forms of testosterone, or methyltestosterone (brand names include Metesto, Methitest, Testred, Oreton Methyl, and Android), are not typically used for women. Testosterone patches like Androderm and Testoderm are also not used for women; however, testosterone patches for women are in development and expected to be available soon. Injectable testosterone is also not recommended for women.

Compounding pharmacies offer testosterone in various forms and strengths for women, including

- Oral capsules
- Gel form, cream form
- Implantable pellets
- Sublingual pills or drops
- Troches

Testosterone is not available in the United States in any form without a prescription.

As far as safety issues are concerned, there is little information regarding the long-term safety of testosterone for women.

Some practitioners believe that testosterone supplementation can help perimenopausal women by improving sex drive, arousal, and orgasmic response, reducing fatigue, and helping aid weight loss by building muscle.

Side effects related to testosterone use in women include:

- Acne
- Hair loss
- Facial hair, including male pattern hair loss
- Deepening voice
- Oilier skin
- Reduced high-density lipoprotein (HDL, "good" cholesterol) levels, raised low-density lipoprotein (LDL, "bad" cholesterol)

Keep in mind that the dose of testosterone for women is small, and side effects are most often associated with too high a dose. For women, generally, the dosage is no more than about one-tenth of what is used in men. Testosterone is not particularly effective in women as an oral drug, so it is best prescribed as a topical gel or cream or as a sublingual.

ESTROGENS

The most commonly prescribed form of estrogen therapy is the category of drugs known as conjugated estrogens. Conjugated estrogens are a mixture of several different estrogens: estrone plus two estrogens found in horses, equilin and equilenin. One type uses horse estrogens derived from horse urine and is known as conjugated equine estrogen. The oral form of this drug is most commonly known by the brand name Premarin. Premarin is also available as a vaginal cream.

There are several oral conjugated estrogen drugs that are synthetically formulated to match the mix in conjugated equine estrogen. These include Cenestin, Congest, C.E.S., and Enjuvia.

Another category of estrogen therapy is oral mixed estrogen formulations known as esterified estrogens (brand names Menest and Estratab) and estropipate/estrone (brand name Ortho-Est).

A form of estrogen, 17-beta estradiol, is designed to replicate human estradiol. Estradiol is available in a number of manufactured forms:

- **Oral estradiol:** Estrace, Femtrace, and generics
- **Estradiol patches:** Estraderm, Alora, Climara, Esclim, Menostar, Vivelle, and Vivelle-Dot; generic estradiol gel/ transdermal: Estro Gel, Elestrin, and Divigel
- **Estradiol topical lotion/transdermal:** Estrasorb
- **Estradiol transdermal spray mist:** Evamist
- **Estradiol vaginal cream:** Estrace Vaginal Cream
- **Estradiol vaginal ring:** Estring, Femring
- **Estradiol vaginal tablets:** Vagifem

Compounding pharmacies offer a variety of forms of estrogen.

Bi-est is a mixture of bioidentical versions of estriol and 17-beta estradiol, usually 90 percent estriol and 10 percent estradiol, or 80 percent estriol and 20 percent estradiol.

Tri-est is a mixture of bioidentical versions of all three key estrogens, usually in the following ratio:

- **Estriol:** 80 percent
- **Estrone:** 10 per cent
- **17-beta estradiol:** 10 percent

Some practitioners customize the percentages of Bi-est or Tri-est, based on a patient's blood or saliva test results.

These compounded estrogens are typically available in different forms from a compounding pharmacy:

- **Oral capsules**
- **Transdermal creams**
- **Vaginal creams**
- **Vaginal suppositories**

- Sublingual pills
- Troches
- Implantable pellets

Wyeth Pharmaceuticals, the manufacturer of Premarin and Prempro, is also in the process of seeking approval for Aprela, a drug designed for postmenopausal women that combines conjugated estrogen with bazedoxifene, a selective estrogen receptor modulator drug to prevent/treat osteoporosis. (Wyeth has been trying to get approval to sell a bazedoxifene-only osteoporosis drug, known as Viviant, for several years, but to date, the FDA has not approved the drug, asking for additional data on blood clots and strokes that appear to be linked to the medication.) According to preliminary studies of Aprela, it may help reduce hot flashes and sleep disruptions, without causing breast tenderness. A two-year study did not find an increase in breast cancer incidence, but given that breast cancer can take a decade to develop, this is not conclusive and requires longer-term research.

There are no forms of estrogen available without a prescription in the United States.

When it comes to estrogen supplementation, it's important to keep in mind that women who have a uterus and are prescribed estrogen treatment also need to be prescribed a progestogen. This helps prevent buildup of the uterine lining (endometrial hyperplasia), which is a side effect of estrogen therapy and a risk factor for uterine cancer. Postmenopausal women who do not have a uterus can be prescribed estrogen without an opposing progestogen. Women who are prescribed a low dose of a vaginal form of estrogen may not require opposing progestogen.

As far as safety is concerned, some doctors point to the fact that estrogen therapy is really the only form of reproductive hormone replacement for women that has been studied fairly extensively. Even then, the results of studies have been confusing, and often contradictory, leaving women—and their doctors—quite confused about the benefits and risks associated with estrogen therapy. I'll attempt to sum up the latest thinking on the pros and cons of estrogen therapy.

Specifically, estrogen therapy—with or without the use of a progestogen—is considered the most effective treatment for several menopause-related symptoms, including

– Vasomotor symptoms, such as hot flashes and night sweats

– Vaginal/urethra atrophy, which can cause dryness, painful intercourse, vaginal infections, and urge incontinence. (Note: While oral estrogen treatment can be prescribed for both vasomotor and vaginal symptoms, for women who only have vaginal symptoms, a vaginal form of estrogen (that is, a gel or a cream) is typically recommended, rather than systemic oral estrogen.)

– Vaginal estrogen treatment has been shown to be effective in helping reduce recurrent urinary tract infections that result from menopausal changes.

– Estrogen helps bone density and reduces the risk of osteoporosis, but it is only effective when the medication is being taken, and the effect does not continue after therapy stops. So using hormone therapy for an extended period to prevent bone loss and to treat serious osteoporosis introduces risks and is typically considered only after other options—bisphosphonate drugs like Fosamax, Boniva, Actonel, Zometa, and raloxifene (Evista)—have failed.

The North American Menopause Society (NAMS) says that if hormone therapy is going to be used, it should be implemented around the time of menopause to treat menopause-related symptoms. NAMS recommends that the lowest effective dose of medication be prescribed, and only for the shortest time necessary to relieve symptoms. When hormone therapy is used, NAMS recommends FDA-approved manufactured medications be prescribed instead of unregulated medications prepared by compounding pharmacies.

Hormones carry risks and side effects. One aspect is especially clear: for women over age sixty who went through a natural menopause and have not been on hormone therapy, doctors do not recommend hormone therapy, because it substantially increases the risk of blood clots, stroke, heart disease, heart attack, breast cancer, and dementia.

For younger women in perimenopause or recently menopausal, there are also risks to estrogen therapy.

- There is a slightly increased risk for stroke.

- Oral estrogen slightly increases the risk of blood clot in the legs (deep vein, or venous, thrombosis [DVT]) and lungs (pulmonary embolism). This does not appear to be the case with transdermal estrogen.

- There is a slightly increased risk of breast cancer. This risk appears to be much lower for short-term use of estrogen and increases with five or more years of estrogen therapy.

- Conjugated equine estrogen is linked to an increased risk in benign breast disease, a condition associated with breast cancer. Estrogen therapy also increases the frequency of abnormal mammograms and the need for diagnostic breast biopsies.

- Estrogen therapy in any woman who has a uterus increases the risk of endometrial hyperplasia and uterine cancer. (Doctors therefore recommend use of a progestogen along with estrogen in women who still have a uterus, to help prevent this buildup and reduce the risk.)

- Women who use estrogen are more likely to have symptomatic gallstones and gallbladder disease.

- There is a slight increase in the risk of ovarian cancer. (But because this cancer is quite rare, the overall risk is still very low.)

- While clot, stroke, and heart attack risks, as well as the health benefits and symptom relief, disappear, a slightly higher risk for breast cancer continues for at least three years after stopping hormone therapy. (The risk is small, however, and translates to about a 0.3 percent extra annual risk for each woman, or three additional cases of breast cancer a year for every 1,000 women taking hormone therapy.)

- Oral estrogen therapy may worsen or provoke stress incontinence.

Interestingly, research released in 2008 suggested that hormone therapy may actually reduce the risk of breast cancer in a very specific group—postmenopausal women who have the *BRCA1* (breast cancer type 1, early onset) genetic mutation—by as much as 42 percent. (The *BRCA1* and *BRCA2* [breast cancer type 2, susceptibility protein] genetic mutations increase a woman's chance of developing breast cancer by as much as 40 to 60 percent, and approximately 3 percent of invasive breast cancers can be attributed to a mutation in *BRCA1* or *BRCA2*.) This study provided interesting results, but experts say that it doesn't offer enough information upon which to base decisions for patients.

Side effects, which are more common with oral estrogen and less common with the topical forms, include

- Headaches, migraines
- Nausea
- Vaginal discharge
- Fluid retention, bloating
- Weight gain
- Breast tenderness
- Spotting or darkening of the skin, particularly on the face (melasma)
- Growth of preexisting uterine fibroids
- Worsening of endometriosis

For some women, side effects may go away after a few weeks of use or are dose-dependent.

More on the pros and cons of estrogen therapy is discussed later in this chapter.

Hormone Combinations

The combination of conjugated equine estrogen and medroxyprogesterone is available by prescription in two different pills: Prempro, which has a fixed estrogen/medroxyprogesterone ratio, and Premphase, which introduces the medroxyprogesterone for the last two weeks of each cycle, to mimic the normal hormonal fluctuations seen in the menstrual cycle.

A particular formulation of estradiol known as ethinyl estradiol is the most common estrogen ingredient in oral contraceptive pills. It is typically combined with various synthesized progestins in the birth control pill. Some common brands are Yasmin, Orthocept, Ortho Tricyclen, Ortho Novum, and Yaz.

Ethinyl estradiol is also combined with the progestin norethindrone in a lower-dose pill used for hormone treatment, Femhrt.

There are a number of oral combinations of 17-beta estradiol and progestins, including

- **17-beta estradiol plus norethindrone acetate:** Activella
- **17-beta estradiol plus drospirenone:** Angeliq
- **17-beta estradiol plus norgestimate:** Prefest

There are also two transdermal patches offering the combination of hormones:

- **17-beta estradiol plus norethindrone acetate:** CombiPatch
- **17-beta estradiol plus levonorgestrel:** Climara Pro

Compounding pharmacies can compound combinations of 17-beta estradiol and natural progesterone.

An oral manufactured drug, Estratest, combines esterified estrogen and methyltestosterone. There is also a generic for this drug.

Compounding pharmacies can also create customized combinations of 17-beta estradiol and testosterone.

For combination therapy, some practitioners are doing what is called "long cycle therapy," in which a low-dose form of estrogen, such as an estrogen patch, is used without accompanying progestin or progesterone. Instead, a dose of a progestogen or progesterone is given every three, six, or twelve months, which will usually trigger bleeding and shedding of the uterine lining and reduce the risk of hyperplasia.

Some doctors are eliminating progestins or progesterone entirely, giving their patients an annual transvaginal ultrasound to look for any thickening of the uterine lining. If the lining doesn't thicken, these practitioners feel that low-dose estrogen without a progestin/progesterone is safe.

A tip: many practitioners recommend that if you still have a uterus and are going to take any form of estrogen (which means you will also need an opposing progestogen to protect the endometrium from buildup), you should first start with the estrogen medication alone, to gauge whether you are getting symptom relief. After eight to twelve weeks, and any dosage adjustments that are necessary for symptom relief, you can add the necessary progestogen. This helps you make a more accurate assessment of the estrogen's effectiveness.

In general, conventional practitioners do not recommend estrogen therapy

- If you suffer from undiagnosed or abnormal genital bleeding
- If you currently have breast cancer or if you have a suspicious lump under evaluation

- If you have a suspected or confirmed estrogen-dependent benign or cancerous tumor or growth
- If you have any history of blood clots in your legs (DVT) or lungs (pulmonary emboli)
- If you have had a stroke or a heart attack in the past year (some physicians say at any point in your medical history)
- If you have any form of liver dysfunction
- If you have a family history of blood clots, strokes, heart disease, breast disease, or cancer
- If you have migraine headaches
- If you have gallbladder disease
- If you smoke

If you do take estrogen or estrogen/progesterone therapy to relieve menopause symptoms, be sure your blood pressure is controlled, and have regular mammograms as recommended by your practitioner.

Hormone Confusion

Why is there so much confusion about hormones?

For the most part, you can blame a study called the Women's Health Initiative (WHI). The WHI was a federally funded study of more than 27,000 women begun in 1991 by the National Institutes of Health (NIH). The objective was to evaluate the effects of hormone treatments on cardiovascular disease, cancer, and osteoporosis.

The most publicized part of the study was the clinical trial of the estrogen-progestin medication Prempro. In July 2002, NIH stopped that trial, announcing that it had become clear to the investigators that the health risks outweighed the benefits. Press conferences were called, and the news media went wild reporting the sound bite that "hormones were dangerous."

What WHI had found was that, in its study population in general, women taking hormones had more heart attacks, strokes, and breast cancer. One especially dramatic finding was that women twenty years or more past menopause taking hormone therapy faced a 28 percent higher risk of heart attack.

Those findings were a surprise to many women and doctors, who had thought that hormones were valuable not only for menopause symptoms, but for prevention of health problems, including heart disease and osteoporosis. Many women were taking hormones just for disease prevention, not for menopausal symptoms.

So the soundbite messages repeated over and over became

- **Hormone therapy is generally not effective for disease prevention and may cause more disease than it prevents.**
- **Hormone therapy is risky, and the dangers outweigh the benefits for women of all ages.**

The frightening and unexpected findings immediately changed the attitude toward hormone therapy, and hormone use understandably plummeted as a result.

In fact, in 2001, before the WHI study findings were released, there were 91 million prescriptions for hormone treatment. From 2001 to 2003, the rate of visits to doctors during which women were prescribed a combination estrogen–progestin hormone therapy dropped by 44 percent. In 2003 there were only 57 million prescriptions written for hormone therapy.

Unfortunately, most people, including doctors, patients, and the media, didn't really understand or look at the specifics of the WHI findings.

Specifically, WHI was flawed in an important way. The average age of women in the WHI was sixty-three, and most of the women studied began taking the hormone medications ten years after their menopause was completed.

So except for a very small cohort of participants, the WHI was not evaluating hormone use in the women most likely to need them—women in their late forties or early fifties in perimenopause or early menopause who are suffering symptoms like hot flashes. Instead, it took a population of women long past menopause and gave them hormone treatment. When the study found that there was little benefit, and in fact significant dangers associated with hormone therapy for this group of older women, the media, many doctors, and women concluded that these concerns applied to all women.

WHI was not designed to understand the risk and benefits of hormone therapy for women in perimenopause or who are recently menopausal. But this aspect of the WHI did clarify one issue: older women long past menopause should not be prescribed hormones. Tara Parker-Pope, a *New York Times* health columnist and author, explains:

> Thank God it was designed the way it was. Even though it was a mistake, they didn't realize that by including older women, they were able to point out the problems with hormones. If it had been designed the right way—studying only recently menopausal women—it seems pretty clear they would have seen positive effects and far less risk, and then they might have put everyone on hormones, including 75-year-old women, without realizing the longer-term dangers.

Women who have had a hysterectomy and don't have a uterus are a unique group. Because they don't require a progestogen and only used estrogen treatment, they actually had lower risk of heart attack and breast cancer and a slightly increased risk of stroke and blood clots. The researchers concluded that this group could take estrogen for up to seven years without raising their risk of breast cancer.

There was a small group of younger women in the study (women of perimenopausal/menopausal age) and interestingly, among that group, the WHI found that hormone therapy actually reduced the risk of heart problems by as much as 24 percent. Overall, hormone users ages fifty to fifty-nine had a 30 percent lower risk of dying of any cause during the five to seven years of the WHI study versus those given a placebo. The women also had fewer hip fractures and a lower risk of colon cancer.

There was, however, a slightly increased risk of clotting and stroke, and a slightly increased breast cancer risk in the younger group. But the increases were small. To put it in perspective, the typical healthy fifty-year-old woman has a risk of about 2 to 3 percent of being diagnosed with breast cancer within the next five years. If she uses hormones, that risk goes up to around 3 percent. (The WHI did not take into account whether younger women had also taken birth control pills prior to hormones, a factor that may have an effect on the cancer risk and warrants further study.)

That additional risk for breast cancer found by WHI in younger women is up for debate. A 2004 study of nearly 375,000 postmenopausal women found that women who took an estrogen/progesterone combination for less than five years did not have an increased risk of breast cancer. So, at worst, there is a slightly increased risk of breast cancer, but there may actually be no risk if a woman limits hormone use to three to five years.

Overall, however, the WHI showed (and subsequent studies have also shown) that shorter-term use of hormones for symptom relief during the perimenopause/menopause transition is generally safe for most healthy women.

Dr. Risa Kagan, a Berkeley, California, gynecologist, an NAMS-certified menopause practitioner, and a spokesperson for NAMS, explains how things have changed:

> The biggest benefit of the Women's Health Initiative is that before that study was released, we had women taking drugs for preventative reasons, with no evidence of prevention. Now we know that there is no reason for postmenopausal women to be on hormone therapy for the rest of their lives. Now, we are no longer looking at hormone "replacement" therapy . . . HRT. We're getting rid of

the R, and we're focusing on hormone therapy . . . HT. We're not trying to replace hormones, but rather, we're focusing on treating symptoms. The goal is to find a dose that will help a woman function and feel well.

Women are still confused, however. Contradictory studies come out regularly, and proponents of different types of hormones (conventional versus bioidentical versus compounded) frequently cite contradictory information about benefits and risks.

Andrea, a thyroid patient who had a hysterectomy at forty-seven, was suffering from severe hot flashes, and her doctor put her on a low dose of estradiol, which helped. But she did some more reading about estrogen.

I got concerned about taking the estrogen replacement, so I stopped taking the estradiol for about three weeks. The flashes came back and my insomnia was worse, so I started back again about a week ago. Now I don't know what to believe. Does it cause higher risk for breast cancer or not?

Unfortunately, many are in the same situation as Andrea, suffering from symptoms but unsure as to whether or not they can use hormones. It's the fallout resulting from the alarmist way in which the WHI results were announced, and the misinformation and misunderstanding of what the results actually showed. Tara Parker-Pope explains:

Doctors are confused, and women are confused. People are being whipsawed back and forth about hormones—they're good, bad, good for some, bad for others . . . it's all over the place. Most doctors don't have time to sift through the medical literature, and they are also influenced by the news media. What happened with the hormone story, there was this initial terrible report from the WHI in July 2002, and that became the "truth" for a while. Over time, people started looking at this data and realized there were flaws. Eventually, they realized that there were two types of women—women near menopause and women long past menopause, and the risks and benefits were different for each group. Now, I think women are suffering hormone fatigue. There have been so many hormone stories that women think it's easier to not think about it and to just "forget it." There is so much conflicting info that these women think, "It's better to not take a pill." While I agree that it's better to not take a pill if you don't have to, a percentage of women are miserable. For women who are suffering—they're miserable, depressed, having hot flashes, can't sleep—the thing to keep in mind is that just because you're not taking a drug, that doesn't mean that you're not harmed. People only look at the risks/benefits of taking a drug, but you have to also look at the risks/benefits of not taking a drug. If you don't do anything, that's a risk. You need to weigh the risks of your symptoms against the modest risks of hormones. But this process takes time to sift through, and doctors don't have that time.

More information keeps coming. In the largest study of hormone therapy since WHI, in late 2008 Danish researchers also confirmed the heart health benefits of hormone therapy in some younger women. They found that women with a uterus who need to use opposing progesterone had a reduction in their risk of heart disease if they used cyclic combined therapy—therapy that caused menstrual bleeding, or periodic progestin/progesterone (Premphase), or periodic progesterone use. (In the study, continuous hormone replacement therapy, like Prempro, which does not produce menstrual bleeding, increased the risk of heart attacks.) For women without a uterus, transdermal application using a gel or patch was also associated with a lower risk of heart disease. Essentially, this study found no increased risk of heart disease for women taking unopposed estrogen and cyclic combined therapy, and a significantly lower risk was found with transdermal estrogen, versus oral estrogen. It's still an issue that requires further study, but these results are promising.

Bioidentical and Compounded Drugs

Before we look at the issue of bioidentical and compounded hormones, it's important to clarify what the terms *synthetic*, *natural*, and *bioidentical* mean in the context of hormones.

A synthetic hormone is one that has a chemical structure that is different from the hormone in humans. A natural or bioidentical hormone is one that has a chemical structure that is identical to the human hormone.

Do not assume, however, that something coming from a "natural source" is necessarily natural. The hormones in conjugated equine estrogen (like Premarin and Prempro) are derived from horse urine, but they are formulated in a way that makes them very different from human estrogens.

Also, don't assume that because a drug is manufactured by a pharmaceutical company that it's not bioidentical. Some people mistakenly believe that only compounded hormones are bioidentical, but brand name and generic estrogen medications that include estradiol (Estrace, Estrogel, and the various estradiol patches like Climara, Menostar, and Vivelle), as well as the oral micronized progesterone drug Prometrium, for example, are bioidentical.

Proponents of bioidentical hormones suggest that they are safer than the synthetic hormones. The logic is that since the hormones mimic human hormones, they are safer.

Proponents of compounded bioidentical hormones also make many health claims for compounded drugs, including

- Estradiol reduces coronary artery disease.
- Estriol has anticancer effects and helps prevent breast cancer.
- Topical estriol is better than estradiol for vaginal and urinary symptoms.

- Estradiol helps with weight loss; conjugated equine estrogen (Premarin) causes weight gain.
- Estradiol helps the cardiovascular system and doesn't promote clotting when used in cream form; conjugated equine estrogen (Premarin) promotes clotting.
- Estradiol doesn't worsen or trigger migraines; conjugated equine estrogen (Premarin) does.
- Estradiol decreases stress incontinence; conjugated equine estrogen (Premarin) worsens it.
- Estradiol decreases dry eyes; conjugated equine estrogen (Premarin) worsens it.
- Progesterone protects against breast cancer; Provera/progestins promote it.
- Progesterone doesn't affect insulin resistance; Provera/progestins increase it.
- Progesterone helps build bone; Provera/progestins promote bone loss.
- Progesterone helps improve sleep; Provera/progestins decrease sleep quality.

Perhaps the most widely known proponent of compounded bioidentical hormones is actress Suzanne Somers. Somers, who wrote about bioidentical hormones in her book *Ageless: The Naked Truth about Bioidentical Hormones*, calls them "the juice of youth." Her book recommended a way of taking compounded hormones that was created by housewife-turned-author T. S. Wiley. Wiley's theory, called the "Wiley protocol," is based on the idea that compounded, transdermal hormones are totally safe when they are replaced in a natural cycle like the fluctuations of a menstrual cycle. Wiley outlined the approach in her book, *Sex, Lies and Menopause*, and has built a profitable business charging doctors and compounding pharmacies to train and "certify" them in her protocol and its products. She claims that her protocol is safe, and that it can treat and cure any number of conditions and symptoms, but there is limited evidence to support her claims. Wiley is reportedly currently tracking the outcomes and quality of life indicators in a three-year "clinical trial" she is conducting with some doctors following her protocol.

So is there any merit to the various claims about bioidentical—in particular compounded—hormones?

The answer is, we really don't know.

On the plus side, compounded hormones definitely have advantages over conventional drugs, in terms of the flexibility of dosing, the ability to eliminate allergens from formulations, a lower cost in some cases, and treatment options where commercial formulations don't exist, like testosterone treatment for women.

Jacob Teitelbaum, MD, author of *From Fatigued to Fantastic* and an internationally known expert on hormone therapy, is a proponent of using bioidenticals. "If I were a woman," says Dr. Teitelbaum, "I'd be on Bi-est and natural progesterone. It's protective of the heart and doesn't increase breast cancer."

Anecdotal evidence and common sense also suggest that bioidentical or compounded medications are safer and/or better than the synthetic formulations.

Tucson, Arizona–based holistic physician Molly Roberts doesn't necessarily feel that all her patients need hormones. "But when they do, I tend to use the bioidenticals," she says. "My philosophy is that I trust thousands of years of evolution. So the closer I can get to nature, the closer I am to having the body work as well as it can." Dr. Roberts also notes that she sees more signs of inflammation with the synthetic hormones.

Bioidentical hormones, and in some cases compounded hormones, are definitely the choice of most integrative, holistic, and complementary physicians. My own doctor and many doctors whose opinions I respect believe, at minimum, that bioidentical forms of hormones are probably safer for their patients.

But right now, we don't have generally accepted evidence in the form of published studies that compounded hormone medications are safer, more effective, or pose fewer risks than conventional hormone treatment.

Just as there is some evidence that the bioidentical and compounded hormones have some benefits, there is also some evidence of risk.

Tara Parker-Pope cautions women to be wary of claims that "natural" or compounded hormones are somehow better. Says Parker-Pope:

> Those are marketing words. Whenever anyone uses the word *natural*, it's a powerful word that we've come to associate with health and goodness. But it can be a dangerous word, because the notion that natural is safer is misleading. When you listen to people peddling natural remedies, someone is always making money off the message . . . capitalism is at work. People who want to debunk that often aren't believed, like if a drug company says, "That's the same thing that I'm selling." But "natural bioidentical estradiol" is the same as the estradiol patch. People just don't want to believe it. I think there probably are benefits to some of these "natural" products, like "natural progesterone." There's evidence that it may be a better choice, but there are also side effects. Just because it's natural, it's not perfect.

For example, there's the issue that compounded hormones are made from the same or similar bulk ingredients that are used in producing bioidentical manufactured hormones. Trying to claim that compounding is superior to manufacturing becomes muddied.

Also, some experts argue that bioidentical hormones are still a risk, because even a woman's own natural estrogen, produced by her own body, is a risk. The evidence? If a woman menstruates early, has a late menopause, or is never pregnant, she has more menstrual cycles, and it's been shown that the more menstrual cycles a woman has, the higher the risk of breast cancer.

Finally, what seems to be a key issue for many doctors is the fact that almost all the hormone research that has been done has used Premarin and Prempro. So, for those doctors who want peer-reviewed research to back up their decisions, there really isn't a choice besides the "well-studied" Premarin and Prempro.

Alexandria, Virginia–based gynecologist and certified menopause practitioner Donna Hurlock, MD, feels most comfortable using Premarin and Prempro. Says Dr. Hurlock:

> I like to use whatever is tried, tested, and easy to use. We have 60 years of data on Premarin and Prempro, and it has a long track record.

Harriet Hall, MD, who calls herself the "Skepdoc" and writes a blog at Skeptic.com, explains why some doctors prefer to prescribe the most studied drugs, Premarin and Provera. Says Dr. Hall:

> There are hypothetical reasons to think "bioidentical" hormones should be superior to Premarin and Provera. But there are also hypothetical reasons to think that they may be no more effective and no safer. The only way to know for sure is to test them in a properly designed placebo-controlled trial. Until this is done, most of us feel more comfortable with the devil we know than the devil we don't know. Women on Premarin and Provera were more likely to have heart attacks and breast cancer, and there's no reason to think providing [hormone replacement therapy] in other forms won't cause the same problems when we have the same amount of experience with them. Think of how many years we used Premarin and Provera before we recognized the risks.

Many conventional physicians are not opposed to bioidenticals, however, as long as they are the FDA-approved drugs, and not compounded hormones.

Dr. Jan Shifren feels very strongly that women should be using FDA-approved products for hormone treatment.

With those products, you get dose-to-dose consistency, bioavailability, and quality control. If a woman wants bioidentical hormones, terrific! I can give you FDA-approved products like oral or transdermal estradiol, and Prometrium. But ultimately, if a woman wants the simplest, least expensive option, Prempro is easy, and the least expensive, and no one should feel that it's any less effective.

Gynecologist and North American Menopause Society spokesperson Risa Kagan, MD, is also willing to work with manufactured bioidenticals. Says Dr. Kagan:

When women ask for compounded bioidenticals, I try to get them to read reputable information and the Menopause Society's statement on the issue. But I can give them natural micronized Prometrium and estradiol in transdermal gel/patches, which are bioidentical. The key thing is that patients have to realize that there's no data right now to say that this is any safer or better than the conjugated estrogen. Hopefully down the road, there will be more definitive information.

THE WYETH ATTACK

Bioidentical hormones have become a huge issue for pharmaceutical giant Wyeth, the manufacturer of Premarin and Prempro, which are synthetic hormones that are not bioidentical. After stopping Premarin and Prempro back in 2002, many of the women who later returned to hormone therapy, and those who began treatment after the WHI findings were released, increasingly went to bioidentical and compounded hormones, products that are not made by Wyeth. Now still hurting from the 50 percent drop in sales of prescription hormones after the 2002 WHI shock wave, Wyeth appears to have as its goal the elimination of the hormone-compounding business entirely.

At the same time, the proponents of compounded bioidentical hormone replacement therapy (BHRT) have invited scrutiny, by making all sorts of broad health claims about the safety and effectiveness of these products, claims that may be true but so far aren't backed up by sound research.

It's not surprising, then, that Wyeth has been waging an all-out war against compounded hormones and the pharmacists, doctors, consumers, and celebrities who tout them, as well as against anyone who is claiming that bioidenticals are better and/or safer. Wyeth is seeking to eliminate the competition and protect its market share and profits.

So far, Wyeth has managed to get the FDA to prohibit marketing of bioidentical hormones as "better/safer" than synthetic hormones. The FDA basically ruled that as far as marketing claims, "a hormone is a hormone." And, according to the FDA, BHRT is basically just a marketing term; there is no credible scientific evidence to support the claims being made regarding the safety and effectiveness of the compounded hormones. The FDA also said that like the FDA-approved manufactured hormone drugs, the compounded bioidenticals may increase the risk of heart disease, clots, breast cancer, and dementia in some women. So, whether it's made by a drug company or mixed by a compounding pharmacist, the FDA's official position is that the risks and benefits should be considered the same.

Wyeth also managed to convince the FDA to put stricter controls on the use of estriol by compounding pharmacies. The FDA did not go so far as to agree to Wyeth's request that the FDA strictly regulate compounding pharmacies like drug companies. But Wyeth doesn't appear ready to give up its campaign against hormone compounding, and it's a battle likely to continue in years to come.

In Favor of Transdermal Estrogen

There are two reasons women who make the decision to take hormone therapy should consider the transdermal (patch, gel, or cream) delivery forms versus oral estrogen.

First, there's evidence that the transdermal forms of estrogen are safer than oral estrogen. When compared with oral estrogen, transdermal estrogen tends to produce more stable serum estradiol levels, less negative effect on triglycerides, and no alteration in sex hormone–binding globulin (SHBG). Gynecologist and North American Menopause Society spokesperson Jan Shifren, MD, feels that FDA-approved transdermals deserve consideration:

> With oral medications, blood levels bump, but when you go through the skin, you are bypassing the liver. Systemic hormones are associated with venous and thrombolic events and pulmonary emboli. We now have some observational studies that show that transdermal estrogen is safer, and these studies look very good. While a woman with a history of deep vein thrombosis or pulmonary embolism is not a candidate for estrogen therapy, a patient with a risk profile for venous clotting might be able to use transdermal forms of the drug.

According to hormone expert David Brownstein, MD:

> We should not for the most part be giving sex hormones orally. These drugs make a first pass through the liver, where they are metabolized down to the various metabolites that may lead to breast cancer, coagulation problems, and other serious side effects. Transdermal hormones metabolize differently and don't create the same problems.

Oral conjugated equine estrogen (Premarin and Prempro) appears to carry higher risks than other forms of estrogen. The esterified estrogens (Menest and Estratab) and transdermal forms of estradiol appear to have a reduced risk of clotting when compared with the conjugated equine estrogen.

Second, oral estrogen also negatively affects the thyroid. Studies have shown that oral estrogen exerts significant effects on levels of thyroxine (T4), and the effects of transdermal estrogen on thyroid function are minimal.

So even in women who have a normal thyroid, oral estrogen is more likely to negatively affect the thyroid and may in fact be a trigger for hypothyroidism. For those women who already have a thyroid condition, oral estrogen can make it worse.

Dr. Jan Shifren has said that, based on some trials of thyroid function in menopausal women, it's clear that thyroid-binding globulin levels go up with oral estrogens but are not affected by transdermal estrogens. Says Shifren, "Thyroid function may be easier to manage if women are using transdermal estrogen, versus oral estrogen."

According to Dr. Uzzi Reiss, women need to be aware that any time they take estrogen—even estradiol—orally, they are also increasing inflammation. "Taking estrogen doesn't do anything positive to inflammatory thyroid conditions and may aggravate them," says Reiss.

Typically, women who are taking thyroid hormone replacement medication may need a small but clinically important increase in their dosage of thyroid medication if they begin oral estrogen treatment. Some experts have found that up to 40 percent of thyroid patients beginning estrogen treatment for menopause experience a worsening of their thyroid hormone levels.

Generally, it's advised that women on thyroid hormone treatment have comprehensive thyroid hormone levels evaluated no more than twelve weeks after they begin any estrogen therapy, to determine if an increase in thyroid dosage is needed.

Even if blood tests are normal, some physicians suggest that if thyroid symptoms worsen after starting estrogen treatment, patients need to slightly increase the dosage to account for the binding effect on thyroid hormone not measurable in the tests.

Do You Need Hormone Supplementation?

Now that you have an idea of the key sex hormones and the various hormone treatment options available, you need to take a look at whether the risks of hormone treatments outweigh the risks and discomfort of not treating symptoms medically.

The answer is really one that only you can answer, because only you know what you're willing to do—outside the realm of prescription drugs—to relieve or cope with symptoms, and how much you are willing to commit to your quality of life and health in general.

Of course, the most important step is being with a doctor who can partner with you to help make those decisions. But keep in mind that doctors have a range of perspectives when it comes to hormones.

On one end of the spectrum are the growing number of holistic physicians and proponents of bioidentical/compounded hormones, who believe that hormone therapy is part of an antiaging, preventative health approach, and that we should be "replacing" hormones so that every woman has the hormone levels of a twenty- or thirty-year-old.

In a way, these practitioners are shifting back to the "hormones for disease prevention" approach that was driving high levels of hormone use before the WHI study burst the hormone bubble. These practitioners believe that, unlike synthetic hormones, bioidentical, transdermal, and/or compounded hormones eliminate the risks, so BHRT offers only benefits. We simply don't have the research yet that backs up these beliefs, however.

At the other end of the spectrum is the belief by a small percentage of doctors that there is no reason whatsoever to go through *any* menopausal symptoms caused by fluctuating estrogen and progesterone. One gynecologist who had this focus told me that most otherwise healthy women in this age range could benefit by simply staying on the birth control pill. "If you want to have an asymptomatic perimenopause-to-menopause transition," she said, "get on birth control pills, and stay on them until you know you're menopausal." Of course, that's an unconventional perspective, as most doctors believe women shouldn't continue on the pill well into their forties or fifties, when menopause traditionally takes place. But she's right. If you stay on the pill through your forties and into your fifties, you aren't likely to suffer a lot of the symptoms we often go through during perimenopause.

Some holistic practitioners, while not advocating hormones for all women, believe that many more women need hormones than is generally recognized. Hormone expert Dr. Uzzi Reiss feels that many of today's women are chronically hormonally depleted. Says Reiss:

People don't eat properly, they don't breathe well, they're not getting enough sleep . . . they're in chronic stress. And when the body is in survival mode, first the hormones are depleted. If there's a question of survival vs. fertility, the body favors survival. You often can't do much to enhance hormone production, but you can replace the depleted hormones. Many women are depleted and chronically deficient in certain hormones, even though their levels show as normal, because the ranges have actually been downgraded to reflect the whole population's depletion.

The most common, middle-of-the-road perspective among most practitioners, both conventional and holistic, is that women who are experiencing significant symptoms should feel comfortable using hormone treatment for a limited time, to relieve symptoms around the time of menopause.

Hormone expert and holistic physician Dr. David Brownstein says:

When it comes to the decision to take hormones, listen to your body. I see women who feel well when estrogen is lower than normal, and I see women who feel better at higher normal estrogen levels. Every woman has a unique biochemical individuality. Every woman doesn't need hormones, but to make the decision, it's helpful for women to be in tune with their bodies, and listen to how they feel.

Some holistic practitioners would like women to consider alternatives or try to avoid medicalizing the natural process of menopause if possible. Noted holistic physician, herbalist, and midwife Tieraona Low Dog, MD, has some thoughts:

When it comes to making a decision to take prescription hormones, I ask women to ask themselves, "Am I willing to take medications that carry risks, to treat 9 to 12 minutes a day of being hot?" We somehow believe we're not supposed to have hot flashes, we believe we're not supposed to have any symptoms of menopause. That seems as unnatural as telling a 12-year-old that her periods will come like clockwork, that she'll never have a cramp, she'll never have breast tenderness, and if she does, that there is medication to take care of every problem. But as grown women, why are we so willing to accept that any kind of hot flash must be treated?

At the same time, Dr. Low Dog believes that there is a place for hormone treatment:

> Hormones are fine for low doses in the short term. I don't discourage it for women who are really bothered by symptoms or whose life is adversely affected by hot flashes. Hormone therapy is the most effective treatment for hot flashes.

There are, of course, opponents to hormones in general, who believe that we simply don't know enough, and what we do know should be enough to warn us off using hormones.

In an interview at the popular menopause Web site Power-Surge. com, the late women's health advocate Barbara Seaman suggested that the effects of treatment are worse than the symptoms for most women.

> The important thing for many women to keep in mind is that the years in their lives when they feel best really are from about 50 to 70 years old. We get our lives back, we put menstrual periods behind us, why are women afraid of hot flashes? Of the natural cycle? Women do not die from menopause. They might have wished they were dead after all the suffering, but many women

have died from the treatment of menopause—strokes, gallblad-der disease, etc. As I said before, the symptoms are not nearly as dangerous as some of the effects of the treatment for meno-pause.

Seaman is famous for calling the unchecked use of menopause hormones "the greatest experiment ever performed on women," which was also the title of a book she wrote on the topic. Said Sea-man:

> They have been used, in the main, for what doctors and scien-tists hope or believe they can do, not for what they know the products can do. . . . Medical policy on estrogens has been to "shoot first and apologize later." . . . [O]ver the years, hundreds of millions, possibly billions of women, have been lab animals in this unofficial trial. They were not volunteers. They were given no consent forms. And they were put at serious, often devastat-ing risk.

The reality? In our lifetimes, we may have to accept that we're not going to get definitive, universally accepted information on ex-actly how, when, and in what form hormones may benefit us or hurt us. So the best we can do is recognize that the "fountain of youth" theory of hormone replacement is a long way from being proven as safe and effective. At the same time, there's rarely justification to undergo extreme physical and emotional suffering simply to avoid short-term use of hormone therapy.

In the end, we must recognize that until we have better evidence, it's prudent to assume that any hormone therapy carries with it some risks, along with benefits.

chapter 6

Natural Approaches to
PERIMENOPAUSE/ MENOPAUSE

Every human being is the author of his own health or disease.

—*Buddha*

When it comes to treating perimenopausal/menopausal symptoms, can—or should—you bypass prescription medications and instead find effective natural approaches? The answer really depends on the severity of your symptoms, as well as your risk factors.

If your symptoms are not especially severe, you may want to try natural approaches, to see if you get any relief and are able to get symptoms under better control so that they are not interfering with your overall quality of life. If you have issues in your medical history that should make you think twice about prescription hormones (for example, a higher risk of breast cancer), then you also may want to try natural approaches, and evaluate the results, before committing to riskier prescription hormone therapy.

The overriding question is this: are natural approaches effective for perimenopausal/menopausal symptoms? The evidence is mixed.

But in practice, whether due to each woman's individual physiology or the skills of the practitioner, some women do find relief from symptoms using complementary, herbal, and other alternatives. So even though we don't have conclusive evidence proving the effectiveness of some of these approaches, that does not mean you should rule them out.

Natural Supplements

One piece of advice about supplements that I think is important to keep in mind comes from holistic hormone expert Uzzi Reiss, MD. According to Dr. Reiss, we should always try supplements one at a time and give them a few weeks. That way, we can see if the supplements are working or, while rare, if they are causing any side effects.

Ob-gyn and menopause expert Jan Shifren, MD, hasn't seen any studies that show that natural approaches are effective for menopausal symptoms, although she says that women certainly can try them.

> At the end of the day, though they're not FDA-approved or monitored, most natural approaches are probably safer than hormones, or antidepressants like Paxil or Effexor. They may be no more effective than placebo, but they are likely safer than the things I can prescribe. I have no concerns about women trying these products, as long as I've informed them of the data. Typically, if a woman wants to try natural approaches, I say, "Why not give it a try?" I see them three months later, and if it wasn't effective, then they can go to prescription therapy.

As many as half of all American women seek alternative or complementary treatments for menopausal symptoms, but reviews of more than seventy different trials and studies have found little to no improvements using herbs, soy, mind–body techniques, magnets, electrical nerve stimulation, homeopathy, or naturopathy.

The key, however, is that the trials of alternatives are usually quite small, and they do not operate in the same way that herbal and natural treatments are given to women by holistic or naturopathic physicians and practitioners, which may be the real key to success. But in order for researchers to "prove" something is effective enough to recommend, they need larger studies and more data. At the same time, the studies usually don't prove that the therapies don't work at all. It's clear, then, that some—but not all—women experience benefits, but you may need to employ a trial-and-error process to see if natural options are right for you.

MACA

Maca (*Lepidium meyenii*), while not well known, is my favorite natural remedy for perimenopausal/menopausal symptoms in thyroid patients. Since the late 1980s, Viana Muller, PhD, an anthropologist and expert in South American medicinal herbs, has been making rain forest herb collecting and study trips to the Amazon river basin and the high Andes of Peru. Since that time, Dr. Muller has single-handedly championed American interest in maca, a vegetable grown in South America.

Maca is a cruciferous root from the same botanical family as the turnip and broccoli. It grows at 12,500 to 14,500 feet above sea level in the high Andean plateaus of central Peru and is the highest growing food plant in the world. It is believed to be one of the earliest domesticated food plants of Peru, along with the potato.

For centuries maca has been used by the native people of Peru as a highly nutritional food, as well as a remedy for hormone issues like fertility, sex drive, premenstrual syndrome (PMS), and menopausal symptoms. It is rich in essential minerals, especially selenium, calcium, magnesium, and iron, and includes fatty acids, such as linolenic, palmitic, and oleic acids, as well as polysaccharides. Maca is an adaptogen, which means it does not increase or decrease hormone levels, but rather helps the hormonal system adapt and balance itself.

Dr. Muller has been actively involved in researching, growing, harvesting, propagating, and distributing a specialized organic and wild-crafted form of maca known as Royal Maca. According to Dr. Muller, native medicine practitioners and herbalists specifically recommend Royal Maca to

- Reduce or eliminate menopausal symptoms, such as hot flashes, vaginal dryness, and hormone-related depression, as an alternative to prescription hormone therapy
- Provide nutritional support for the endocrine system, including the adrenals, the thyroid, and the ovaries (also the testes)
- Regulate and normalize menstrual cycles
- Promote healthy fertility in both women and men
- Promote healthy libido and erectile function
- Support a healthy immune system without overstimulating the immune system or endangering people with autoimmune disease
- Increase energy, stamina, and endurance

Royal Maca appears to work through the pituitary, helping to balance all of the endocrine and reproductive glands. Says Dr. Muller:

The alkaloids in the maca root stimulate the hypothalamus and pituitary to produce more precursor hormones, which then impact all of the endocrine glands—the pineal, adrenals, ovaries, testes, pancreas, and thyroid gland. So maca appears to be stimulating the body to produce its own hormones more adequately rather than supplying hormones from an outside source.

Maca also appears to have an adaptogenic effect on the immune system, without stimulating the immune system. Research has shown that maca works in an entirely different way than plant hormones/phytoestrogenic herbs/isoflavones like soy, black cohosh, and red clover. Instead, its action relies on plant sterols, which act as chemical triggers to help the body itself produce a higher level of hormones appropriate to the age and gender of the person taking it.

Royal Maca also reportedly helps with thyroid function for people with Hashimoto's disease and hypothyroidism. According to Dr. Muller:

> I was surprised to receive feedback from hundreds of women with hypothyroid issues who have benefited from taking Royal Maca. Most of them were having other hormonal imbalances, such as PMS, perimenopausal or menopausal symptoms and discovered "accidentally" how much better they felt when combining Royal Maca with their thyroid medication.

Since introducing maca to the United States in the 1990s, Dr. Muller has seen a dramatic increase in the use of this medicinal herb by holistic practitioners. She has also personally worked with many women who have used Royal Maca for perimenopausal/menopausal symptoms, hypothyroidism, or both.

The Specifics on Royal Maca

Typically, to support the thyroid, Dr. Muller recommends taking one or two Royal Maca capsules daily with breakfast. (She also does not recommend taking Royal Maca along with prescription hormone therapy, like estrogen.) Some women are concerned that maca, being a cruciferous, goitrogenic root vegetable, could slow down the thyroid. But the precooking process in preparing Royal Maca capsules removes the goitrogenic properties, and there are no reports of goiter promotion from maca usage.

According to Dr. Muller, combining Royal Maca with other hormonal treatments can worsen hot flashes, irritability, sleeplessness, or headaches. Women who want to take maca for perimenopausal/menopausal symptoms should, therefore, not take prescription estrogen treatments, estrogenic herbs like black cohosh and red clover, hormone precursors like pregnenolone, human growth hormone (HGH), soy isoflavone supplements, or adaptogenic treatments like ginseng. Dr. Muller recommends that women wait at least four weeks after taking these medications or treatments before beginning maca. She says that progesterone does not need to be stopped, but that women may find they need less, or can even stop it.

For women who are suffering from perimenopausal/menopausal symptoms who are not taking any prescription estrogen or phytoestrogen supplements, Dr. Muller recommends that you start with one capsule a day (or two, if symptoms are especially acute). After a week, gauge your symptoms; if they're not substantially better, add a capsule. When you feel that your symptoms are about 80 percent improved, you should remain at that dose, because Royal Maca typically has a cumulative effect over time.

If you go off prescription hormones to start maca, Dr. Muller recommends going "cold turkey." According to Muller:

If you had hot flashes before you started taking hormones, they will probably return. So after two weeks of taking nothing, you can start taking one capsule a day of Royal Maca. At the beginning of the fourth week, you can take two capsules a day. You will probably continue to experience your hot flashes, however. After four weeks of no hormones, you can increase your dosage of Royal Maca as follows. If your hot flashes are mild (1 or 2 a day), take 3 caps a day. If your hot flashes are moderate (3 to 5 a day or night sweats), you can start with 4 a day. Evaluate after a week. Increase to 6 capsules daily if your hot flashes are not 80% better. If your hot flashes are severe (more than 6 daily and frequent night sweats), start with 6 capsules a day for 5 days. Then, if necessary, increase to 9 a day for another 5 days.

According to Dr. Muller, some women may need even more, but at that point, they may might take 2 teaspoons of Royal Maca powder daily, because it's more economical. (One teaspoon of powder equals six capsules.)

(Note: Women who are petite or highly sensitive to small amounts of herbs or pharmaceutical drugs should typically cut the dosage in half.)

Another formulation of Royal Maca adds diindolylmethane (DIM). DIM is a compound from plants that can help shift the balance of sex hormones; in particular, it helps stimulate more efficient estrogen metabolism. This allows estrogen to be broken down, or metabolized, into good estrogen metabolites, rather than the forms of estrogen that are responsible for cancer. When estrogen metabolizes too slowly, or metabolizes to "bad" estrogens, women can suffer from breast pain and tenderness. Dr. Muller recommends Royal Maca with DIM for women who have symptoms that suggest inflammation or who have had problems with periods, ovarian cysts, or fibroid tumors.

Maca is considered very safe and rarely has side effects. In a woman taking regular Royal Maca, side effects including breast tenderness, insomnia, jitteriness, and slight depression may indicate some estrogen dominance, in which case the formulation with DIM may help. If the original symptoms return, that may be a sign that a woman has gotten too high a dose and needs to cut back slightly.

As for long-term safety concerns, various clinical trials and animal studies have not found any evidence of adverse reactions or toxicity. As a food product in use for centuries, experts believe that maca has a low potential for toxicity. Studies have not been done, however, that demonstrate the long-term safety in women. Very rarely are people allergic or sensitive to maca. One caution, however: Dr. Muller does not recommend that women with estrogen-dependent cancers or who are on any estrogen-blocking drugs, like tamoxifen, use maca.

It's important to be aware that low-cost and mass-produced maca may be grown in areas outside the high Andean plateau, cultivated using chemical fertilizers and pesticides, and heat-processed in nontraditional ways that make it ineffective.

My Own Story

In my own case, I took Royal Maca periodically in early perimenopause, because my cycles were becoming shorter and my periods were coming more frequently. After I started taking Royal Maca, I found that my periods weren't coming as frequently and that the cycles normalized for quite a while.

Later into my perimenopause, my cycles became classically unpredictable, with long gaps (as much as forty to sixty days) between each period. This is also when I started to develop hot flashes. I did not have what I consider severe hot flashes: I usually had two or three a day, more often in the evening around bedtime. (But I was not waking up with night sweats, and I didn't have rapid heartbeat or other issues associated with hot flashes.) Remembering how Royal Maca had worked to help regulate my periods, I started taking it again. Much to my surprise, within a few days, my hot flashes stopped. As I go to press, I am still in perimenopause, and I am still on Royal Maca. (I've been able to get hot flash relief at two capsules a day, but to avoid breast tenderness I was getting as a side effect, I eventually switched to the Royal Maca with DIM.)

MELATONIN

Many women are aware of the benefits of melatonin as a sleep aid, but what you may not realize is that melatonin can have powerful hormonal effects for women in perimenopause and menopause.

Melatonin is a hormone produced by the pineal gland, which is located in the brain. The pineal is the master controller of our body's clock, including our day-to-day circadian clock that tells us when to sleep and when to wake and the biological clock that decides on bigger hormonal issues, such as when we enter puberty and menopause.

The pineal gland controls the circadian rhythm—our daily cycle of sleeping and waking—by releasing a hormone called melatonin, produced primarily at night. Melatonin synthesis and release are stimulated by darkness.

The pineal also contains thyrotropin-releasing hormone (TRH), which the pineal uses to tell the pituitary to produce thyroid-stimulating hormone (TSH). Melatonin is also apparently instrumental in the breakdown of thyroxine (T4) into triiodothyronine (T3), creating heat and energy.

Based on its role in circadian rhythm and sleep, melatonin has become well known as a helpful sleep aid, as a treatment to help prevent jet lag and reset the body clock to a new time zone or to help night shift workers who have difficulty sleeping.

It was as a sleep aid that I first started using melatonin nightly, at one point over a year ago. I had been waking up more frequently and found myself often unable to fall back asleep. Then, when I woke in the morning, I felt fuzzy-brained and tired, even after eight or more hours of sleep. I started taking a low dose of melatonin (3 mg), which I took around 11:00 p.m., about an hour before I usually fell asleep. What I found was that I woke less frequently, and when I did, I was able to turn over and fall back asleep easily. Even better, I was waking up in the morning feeling refreshed and energetic, in a great mood. Even more surprising, I was actually waking up a few minutes before my alarm. (This is definitely not characteristic, as I typically was one of those people who hit the snooze bar multiple times, and only then begrudgingly dragged myself grumpily out of bed. So waking before the alarm and feeling great was quite uncommon.)

When I started taking melatonin, I was also well into what I thought was menopause. My last period had been more than five months earlier, and even before then, they'd become erratic again. I had weathered a period of hot flashes (using the maca, as mentioned earlier), and the hot flashes were gone. I'd seen my physician, who found that I had extremely high levels of follicle-stimulating hormone (FSH) and luteinizing hormone (LH)—markers that can confirm menopause in a woman who isn't having any more periods—and my estrogen and progesterone levels were low. So my doctor and I both assumed that I was in menopause; all I needed was to go the full twelve months without a period, and it would be official. And so what happened next surprised me.

About two months after I started taking melatonin, my periods came back. And when they came back, they were very normal. They weren't unusually heavy, as they had been before. The color was red, not brown, as they had been six months earlier. And, perhaps most surprising of all, they started coming regularly every twenty-eight days.

I didn't immediately connect the melatonin with the return of a normal menstrual cycle. But with nothing else changed in my regimen, I had to wonder if a normalized menstrual cycle in perimenopausal/menopausal women was a known side effect of melatonin. I delved into the research. That's when I discovered Dr. Walter Pierpaoli and his ground-breaking research on melatonin.

Melatonin and Our Hormones

Walter Pierpaoli, MD, created a sensation back in 1996 with the release of his book, *The Melatonin Miracle: Nature's Age-Reversing, Disease-Fighting, Sex-Enhancing Hormone*. The book was a bestseller, and Dr. Pierpaoli's *Melatonin Miracle* introduced Americans to melatonin, which had just become available over the counter in the United States a few years earlier, and its roles as sleep aid, jet lag remedy, immune enhancer, antioxidant cancer fighter, stress reducer, and cure for low libido.

But the book was not a one-time effort by Dr. Pierpaoli. For decades, he has been researching and studying melatonin and its effects, and he continues to do so today.

I had the opportunity to read Dr. Pierpaoli's book, as well as an article in the December 2005 *Annals of the New York Academy of Sciences*, which was titled "Reversal of Aging: Resetting the Pineal Clock." This edition of the *Annals* featured numerous articles and research findings related to melatonin, including several reports from Dr. Pierpaoli. I also had the pleasure to speak with Dr. Pierpaoli personally, to learn more about his ideas about melatonin and reproductive and thyroid hormones.

In all this research, I learned that melatonin is much more than a sleep aid. Rather, the pineal gland controls our body clock, and its chief product, melatonin, is not a classic hormone, like endocrine hormones, but more of a chemical mediator that operates in ways we don't completely understand, but that Dr. Pierpaoli is extensively studying.

What Dr. Pierpaoli explains in his book and research findings is that the pineal gland produces less and less melatonin as we age, but if melatonin supplements are taken when levels are naturally declining, some of the effects of aging can be slowed, stopped, or even, says Dr. Pierpaoli, reversed. Dr. Pierpaoli also has found that melatonin can resynchronize not only the circadian rhythms of the wake–sleep cycles, but the endocrine system overall.

Dr. Pierpaoli believes that providing supplemental melatonin, in a dose of 3 mg nightly, allows the pineal gland to "rest," so to speak, and protects it from aging, which then slows down the aging process for other glands and organs. It's a controversial theory, but Dr. Pierpaoli and others have conducted some intriguing studies that suggest he is on to something.

Animal studies conducted by Dr. Pierpaoli found that older animals treated with melatonin returned to normal daily cycling of thyroid hormones. Mice who were twenty-four months old and treated with melatonin (twenty-four months is the mouse equivalent of seventy-five years for humans) had ovaries that were double the size of untreated mice, suggesting more youthful sexual function. Dr. Pierpaoli also transplanted the pineal glands of aging mice into young mice, and vice versa. The young mice with the old pineal glands developed all sorts of ailments associated with aging, became less vigorous and fertile, and died far younger than normal. The old mice with the young pineal glands regrew hair, gained energy, developed a renewed sex drive, and lived, on average, so long that if they were people, they'd have been energetic, active, healthy, and sexually active well past one hundred years of age.

But what explained my own surprising return of normal menstrual cycles was an Italian study of perimenopausal and menopausal women ages forty-two to sixty-two, evaluating the effects of a daily dose of 3 mg of synthetic melatonin over six months. That study found that the melatonin increased estrogen levels and improved thyroid function. The women under fifty using melatonin also had reduced levels of LH and FSH as a result of the melatonin. In some of the younger women, normal menstrual cyclicity was restored. Surprisingly, a number of women who were already postmenopausal even returned to normal menstrual cycles. Basically, according to Dr. Pierpaoli and his fellow researchers, low-dose melatonin was delaying or, in some cases, apparently reversing characteristic endocrine changes that occur during menopause.

With regard to the thyroid, the melatonin didn't appear to change the TSH levels, but it did help facilitate conversion of T4 to T3, resulting in increased T3 levels. A remarkable 96 percent of women in the study who had taken melatonin also reported total disappearance of morning depression, a symptom that is common in perimenopausal and menopausal women. The women also had fewer complaints about hot flashes, fewer heart palpitations, and better quality and duration of sleep.

While this was not a large study, it was rigorously conducted and suggests that melatonin has a key role in hormonal regulation for perimenopausal and menopausal women, perhaps even more so for those with thyroid imbalances.

Interestingly, the pineal gland may actually be the link that establishes the well-known connection between menstrual cycles and the lunar cycle. (The majority of women menstruate at the new moon, and a woman's highest melatonin levels are typically seen during the dark phase of the moon.) Melatonin also fluctuates with the monthly menstrual cycle.

Dr. Pierpaoli actually believes that the drop in melatonin that takes place in a woman's forties may be the hormonal signal that tells the body to begin the perimenopausal transition. We know that in women from forty to forty-four, melatonin typically declines substantially. Interestingly, this is the point that is often the beginning of perimenopause. The next big significant point of melatonin decline is from fifty to fifty-four years, around the time that the menstrual period finally stops for good in most women.

Dr. Pierpaoli's intriguing theory gained support with the findings of a 2008 study reported in the journal *Menopause*. That study found that the pineal gland, through melatonin, is involved in the mechanisms that regulate the onset of menopause, and by maintaining higher levels of melatonin, the onset of menopause can be delayed.

Dr. Pierpaoli is, without question, a zealous advocate for melatonin. His almost one-hundred-year-old mother-in-law, Emmy, who was diagnosed in her seventies with Parkinson's disease, is still going strong, and Dr. Pierpaoli credits her daily dose of 3 mg of melatonin. Her Parkinson's symptoms disappeared a few years after her diagnosis, also thanks to melatonin, says Dr. Pierpaoli. The doctor himself is a good advertisement for his antiaging approach, in his eighties, energetic, and keeping up a rigorous schedule of activities, research, speaking, writing, and traveling around the world. Dr. Pierpaoli said that if he could go back in time knowing what he knows now, he would have started taking melatonin at around age thirty.

Dr. Pierpaoli maintains that melatonin acts like a hormonal adaptogen, helping to moderate adrenal, thyroid, and reproductive hormones, and maintaining the day–night, monthly, seasonal, and lifetime cyclicity of hormones. He also believes that melatonin increases the density of estrogen receptors in target tissues like the breasts, uterus, and ovaries, and improves their sensitivity.

Some of the other effects of melatonin reported by Dr. Pierpaoli are

- Adaptogenic effects on cortisol levels
- Prevents atrophy of the ovaries, vagina, and uterus
- Extends fertility

- Raises high-density lipoprotein (HDL, "good" cholesterol)
- Lowers blood pressure

Says Dr. Pierpaoli:

Melatonin is not a hormone itself, but truly a "queen of all hormones," which monitors and directs the whole "hormonal orchestra."

OTHER DOCTORS ON MELATONIN

Dr. Pierpaoli is not the only advocate for melatonin in perimenopausal/menopausal women. Noted gynecologist and hormone expert Dr. Uzzi Reiss believes that many of us are suffering from low melatonin levels. Says Dr. Reiss:

We're supposed to wake up with the sunrise, be outside till sunset. Instead, we wake up to a lighted house, we go in to an office with lights, come home and turn on lights. We get less natural light exposure during the day and less darkness at night— both negatively affect melatonin.

Holistic physician Molly Roberts suggests that we consider ways to naturally increase melatonin. Says Dr. Roberts:

We can dim the lights a few hours before bed and turn off the television before it's time to sleep. These ideas may naturally help us raise melatonin levels.

Thyroid and hormone expert David Browstein, MD, feels that melatonin is "incredibly safe" for most patients. Says Brownstein:

Low-dose melatonin can be an incredibly helpful part of hormone balancing. Not only is it useful for sleep, but it's also useful for helping the other hormones, and in particular, improved T4-to-T3 conversion.

Hormone and thyroid expert Richard Shames, MD, feels that melatonin can be useful, but he doesn't necessarily feel that everyone needs the 3 mg dose that Dr. Pierpaoli typically advocates.

You might want to start out with 3 mg, then see if you can get just as good a benefit from going to 2 mg, and then possibly to 1 mg. My general opinion is that a 1 mg dose is not likely to cause headache and depression as a side effect.

Dr. Jacob Teitelbaum, who works with patients with chronic fatigue syndrome, fibromyalgia, and thyroid disease, feels that the effectiveness of melatonin may stem from its ability to promote quality sleep. Says Teitelbaum:

What happens is when you don't have sleep, you're suppressing the whole system. Getting proper sleep is restoring hypothalamic function. And the melatonin is, at minimum, helping ensure better quality of sleep. In addition, in the entire hormone system, the pineal can be viewed as the leader of the whole orchestra. If it's sluggish, the rest of the hormonal system can be sluggish.

Dr. Molly Roberts also feels that melatonin is helpful for sleep in perimenopausal and menopausal women. According to Roberts:

I recommend melatonin on a regular basis. The first symptom of perimenopause is often a problem with sleep. You fall asleep but then wake up in the middle of the night, feeling anxious and stressed out. When you wake, you feel tired. The sleep clock gets out of balance. Melatonin can help. It's not a sleeping pill, but really a way of resetting the sleep clock.

Supplementing with Melatonin

The main side effects from low-dose (5 mg or less) melatonin appears to be some morning grogginess, vivid dreams and nightmares, and a mild headache after use in a small percentage of users. There are rare reports of allergic skin reactions from melatonin supplements.

There really are no published long-term studies evaluating the data regarding use of low-dose melatonin. All the doctors I spoke with, many who use low-dose melatonin themselves and recommend it to patients, felt that, based on the results of shorter-term studies, we are not likely to discover any problems with longer-term use of low-dose melatonin. Melatonin should not be used by women who are pregnant or lactating, however.

If you're interested in supplementing with melatonin, you should choose the brand carefully. You want to be sure you are getting pure, pharmaceutical-grade melatonin. Experts suggest that you use only synthetic melatonin, which carries no risk of transmitting animal brain diseases.

I personally prefer a formulation that Dr. Pierpaoli himself created. (He wanted to make sure there was a pharmaceutical-grade melatonin available without prescription, and his formulation, known as TI-MElatonin, is a 3 mg tablet that also includes zinc, to help potentiate the melatonin, and selenium, for the immune system.) The Life Extension Foundation has also created a good-quality time-released melatonin in 300 mcg (0.3 mg) capsules. These might be helpful for those who find half a 3 mg tablet too high a dose.

You'll sometimes hear that melatonin is not recommended for people with autoimmune disease. For those women who have thyroid problems due to autoimmune Hashimoto's or Graves' disease, this may seem problematic. But it's important to note that the concern was reportedly based on an isolated case where melatonin was linked to autoimmune hepatitis. Dr. Pierpaoli believes that melatonin is helpful for autoimmune diseases and explained why in an interview he gave to International Anti-aging Systems, a U.K.-based pharmacy:

> As for autoimmunity, melatonin must be used in autoimmune diseases simply because it will restore a normal immune reaction and the capacity of the immune system to recognize "self" antigens. We have observed complete recovery! The etiology of all autoimmune diseases affecting the skin, the glands, the blood and any other tissue is based on congenital or acquired inability to recognize our own body tissues and thus to mount an autoimmune reaction. Aging itself is largely a hidden, latent and insidious autoimmune process leading to vasculitis (sclerosis of vessels), autoantibodies and cancer. Our work of 40 years has led to the demonstration that immunity is totally under hormonal control. Melatonin will not increase the synthesis of aggressive autoantibodies; on the contrary it will progressively lead to healing of the basic hormonal derangements underlying and initiating the autoimmune process.

PHYTOESTROGENS

One of the biggest controversies for women in perimenopause/menopause—and for women with thyroid problems—is the use of phytoestrogens, whether in food, herbal, or supplement form, as natural treatment for symptoms like hot flashes.

In order to understand the controversy, let's take a look at the phytoestrogens, what they are, and the risks and potential benefits for women.

A phytoestrogen, which is sometimes called a dietary estrogen or plant estrogen, is a compound found in plants that has some biochemical similarity to estradiol, so that, when consumed, it can have an estrogenic effect. Basically, isoflavones bind to estrogen receptors, and it's thought that by mimicking the effects of estrogen, they may be able to block some of estrogen's negative effects and risks and reduce the risk of hormone-associated cancer.

There are several different phytoestrogens, but the best known are the isoflavone phytoestrogens, including soy and red clover, and the lignans, including flaxseed.

The highest concentrations of phytoestrogens are found in flax-seed, soy products, soy protein concentrate, tofu, and tempeh, followed by

- Sesame seeds
- Multigrain bread
- Millet
- Barley
- Lentils
- Kidney beans
- Lima beans
- Rye
- Red clover

Phytoestrogens have gotten a great deal of attention because they may have antioxidant benefits, as well as cancer- and heart disease–fighting capabilities. In addition, they have a reputation as being a natural option to help with menopausal symptoms such as hot flashes. Studies so far, however, have not supported any of the anticancer claims for phytoestrogens.

Phytoestrogens: Are They Effective?

Soy and red clover, which both contain isoflavone phytoestrogens, are popular for treating menopause. Soy is often recommended to women in its food form—tofu, tempeh, miso, soy milk, edamame, soy burgers, and so on—but also in pills and protein powders that contain high concentrations of the phytoestrogens found in soy, known as isoflavones.

The fact that women in Asian countries, who regularly have soy in their diet, have fewer hot flashes and menopausal symptoms has

frequently been used to justify the belief that soy can treat menopausal symptoms.

Despite the myths that prevail, Asians actually do not eat large
quantities of soy. Rather, the typical Asian diet may include 5 to 10
grams of soy protein per day. This is in contrast to some American
diets that may include as much as 60 grams of soy protein a day,
from various processed forms of soy, soy supplements, soy milk,
and so on.

So far, the proven benefit that soy proponents can offer is that
substituting soy protein for animal protein can slightly reduce cholesterol levels. But can soy foods help hot flashes? The evidence is
mixed. In fact, in eight different randomized controlled trials of soy
foods, only one of the studies found a significant reduction in the
frequency of hot flashes, but several showed a slight reduction in
frequency. Generally, there's little published evidence to support the
idea that increasing soy isoflavone intake from food or supplements
substantially improves hot flashes. At the same time, we know that
Asian women, who traditionally have a higher amount of soy in the
diet, have much lower rates of hot flashes than American women.
And doctors and women themselves continue to report that soy
helps somewhat with hot flashes and menopausal symptoms.

Studies regarding red clover have also been mixed. Most of them
have focused on a popular over-the-counter menopause supplement,
Promensil, that includes 40 grams of isoflavones per capsule. One
study found that, at the daily dosage of one 40 mg tablet, Promensil
(a preparation of red clover) had no effect on symptoms, but there
was a slight reduction in moderate to severe symptoms at 80 mg per
day. Numerous other studies on Promensil and other red clover formulations have shown no effect on menopausal symptoms.

Flaxseeds contain high levels of omega-3 fatty acids, as well as
lignan phytoestrogens. Apart from the phytoestrogen properties, flax
is thought to stabilize blood sugar and function as a laxative (due to
its high fiber content). Some studies have shown a slight reduction in

menopausal symptoms in women using flaxseed compared with a placebo, but it's not considered enough to be statistically significant.

The reality is that with some natural approaches, we simply don't have widespread, long-term research studies that give definitive information. When we do have studies that show benefits to natural approaches, the results are sometimes reported to be "not statistically significant."

What this means is that there isn't statistical evidence to back up observations of an impact. It doesn't discount entirely the possibility of a cause–effect connection.

Keep in mind that failing to find statistical evidence of a relationship doesn't prove there isn't one.

Some experts suggest, for example, that factors that are not obvious to researchers may make some women more predisposed than others to respond well to natural treatments. Regarding phytoestrogens, for example, a 2005 study on menopause from the journal *Human Reproduction Update* said:

> Recent data suggest that only individuals capable of metabolizing isoflavone daidzein into equol may receive significant health benefits, and thus populations must be analyzed separately by microflora and metabolic characteristics. Significant results are likely to be obscured when subpopulations are analyzed together, particularly in those studies carried out among Western populations in which only approximately 30% are equol producers compared to Japanese populations where 50–60% of menopausal women are equol producers.

Nationally known nutritionist Ann Louise Gittleman, PhD, author of the popular *Fat Flush Plan*, has found that for many women, soy is problematic because it's a hidden food allergen. Also, Dr. Gittleman finds that soy isoflavones work with people who are copper deficient or copper balanced but not in people who have excess copper. Dr. Gittleman talks at great length about the effects of excess copper, a problem that she has found is especially common in peri-menopause/menopause, and in thyroid patients, in her terrific book, *Why Am I Always So Tired?*

Holistic physician Tieraona Low Dog, MD, says that soy appears to work only for a subsection of her patients.

Some women do well with soy, some don't. Some can convert it into active compounds, others can't. I've found that vegetarians may be better able to convert soy. But in general, I haven't found soy overly helpful for the majority of women.

Taking Phytoestrogens

In general, if you are interested in trying phytoestrogens for menopause symptoms, most of the experts I interviewed agreed that you should bypass supplement forms and focus on incorporating them into your diet. That means you probably can give a pass to red clover supplements like Promensil and any isoflavones or phytoestrogen supplements that come in a bottle.

Holistic nutritionists Dr. Annemarie Colbin and Dr. Ann Louise Gittleman both recommend that perimenopausal/menopausal women who want to incorporate flax in their diet grind flaxseeds and add them to foods like cereals, oatmeal, soups, and salads. Keep in mind that flax is high in fiber, so you may want to introduce it gradually.

Also, remember that you will want to have your thyroid re-checked six to twelve weeks after starting or stopping any dietary changes that include fiber (including flaxseeds).

If you are going to eat soy, most of the experts I spoke with agreed: stay away from processed forms of soy, and stick to soy in its natural, fermented forms, such as tempeh and miso. Dr. Ann Louise Gittleman has some thoughts:

Make sure the soy is not genetically modified, and that it's served in its original form, the Asian way, and fermented—like tofu or tempeh or miso.

Dr. Annemarie Colbin thinks soy may be oversold. Says Colbin:

I find it interesting that there's such a push for soy as a health food ever since soybeans became genetically engineered. These big companies have a huge marketing machine. I would not use any of the imitation meat soy foods, or any soy that is extruded, extracted, or genetically engineered. Just miso, a little tofu, tempeh occasionally. I have heard of women finding soy milk helpful for hot flashes, so you can occasionally try a glass of soy milk or a little tofu. But two times a week at most.

Dr. Jacob Teitelbaum feels that for women suffering hot flashes, they can try soy—in moderation—and see if it helps.

I'd suggest a woman consider trying a small bit of soy every day—like a handful of edamame, or some soy milk or soy cheese.

I think that holistic physician Molly Roberts summed it up well. According to Dr. Roberts, "Soy is one of those things where it's important to remember: everything in moderation—a little goes a long way."

Safety

In the short term, the various phytoestrogens appear to be safe, with few adverse effects. There are no studies, however, demonstrating the safety of longer-term use of high-dose phytoestrogens.

With any of the phytoestrogens, there is a question of the impact on hormone-sensitive tissue and the potential to cause or aggravate hormone-sensitive cancers. So far, we do not have information that shows that long-term use of phytoestrogens is safe in this respect.

In fact, there are some concerns, especially regarding the risk of endometrial hyperplasia (a buildup of the uterine lining, which may precede cancer) in women using high levels of soy extract. Many practitioners caution against use of soy and other phytoestrogens—except as an occasional food—for certain groups of women, especially

- Women who have had or are at increased risk for cancers of the breast, uterus, and ovaries
- Women who have had uterine fibroids
- Women taking birth control pills and prescription hormone therapy
- Women taking cancer drugs known as selective estrogen receptor modulators (SERMs), such as tamoxifen

Gynecologist and North American Menopause Society spokesperson Dr. Risa Kagan explains why women should be cautious about soy as a menopause treatment:

I think there is confusion about soy. To take excessive amounts of soy is controversial; what are the proven benefits? There may be some benefits for heart-healthy diet, but to indulge in high levels of phytoestrogens, thinking it's healthy, is questionable. We're telling breast cancer patients to be careful about how much soy to consume, because we don't know the effects. It's one thing for women to grow up in Asia, eating a particular diet, but for older Western patients with a breast cancer risk, we really don't know the impact of a diet heavy in soy protein.

The isoflavones in soy are considered endocrine disrupters and have the ability to disturb proper thyroid function. Much like they do with estrogen, isoflavones can fit into the body's thyroid receptor sites, where they contribute to functional hypothyroidism at the cellular level, due to their receptor-blocking capabilities.

There are concerns about the impact on the thyroid of overconsumption of phytoestrogens, soy in particular. One study involving premenopausal women gave them 60 grams of soy protein per day for one month. This amount was enough to disrupt the menstrual cycle, and the effects continued for three months after the soy was eliminated from the diet.

Another study found that intake of soy over a long period causes enlargement of the thyroid and suppresses thyroid function. Other studies have shown that high soy intake in premenopausal women could suppress ovarian production of estradiol and progesterone by as much as 20 to 50 percent.

In a February 18, 1999, official letter of protest to the Food and Drug Administration (FDA), Doerge and Daniel Sheehan, who at that time were the FDA's two key experts on soy, protested the health claims approved by the adminstration on soy products, saying:

> There is abundant evidence that some of the isoflavones found in soy, including genistein and equol, a metabolize of daidzen, demonstrate toxicity in estrogen sensitive tissues and in the thyroid. This is true for a number of species, including humans. Additionally, isoflavones are inhibitors of the thyroid peroxidase, which makes T3 and T4. Inhibition can be expected to generate thyroid abnormalities, including goiter and autoimmune thyroiditis. There exists a significant body of animal data that demonstrates goitrogenic and even carcinogenic effects of soy products. Moreover, there are significant reports of goitrogenic effects from soy consumption in human infants and adults.

The argument about soy's dangers to the thyroid continues, with spokespeople from the soy industry arguing that it is safe and has no effect on the thyroid, and other researchers periodically releasing studies that show that phytoestrogens have endocrine-disrupting, thyroid-slowing capabilities. For thyroid patients, however, it appears that the isoflavone-intensive forms of soy (for example, supplements and powders) may be more problematic, while occasional use of a fermented soy food may not pose a danger. But overconsumption of phytoestrogens may in fact be a trigger for thyroid disease in some women and may worsen thyroid problems in women who already have a thyroid condition.

To sum up, then, when used in moderation as foods (that is, fermented forms of soy and flaxseeds) and not overconsumed, phytoestrogens appear to be safe.

Will they help your menopause symptoms? Possibly. You have to try them to find out.

Is it safe to use phytoestrogens regularly and over a longer period of time, to help resolve your menopausal symptoms? There, you need to be careful. When overconsumed or taken in high-concentration dietary supplements over longer periods of time, phytoestrogens may be associated with thyroid dysfunction, thickening of the uterus, and other hormonal effects. The risk that phytoestrogens will stimulate certain forms of estrogen receptor-positive cancers, including breast and uterine cancer, is still a question that has not been resolved.

Other Supplements

BLACK COHOSH

Black cohosh (*Actaea racemosa*) is one of the best-known herbs used as a perimenopause/menopause treatment. It's a perennial plant, native to North America. It was used by Native American healers and doctors for centuries to help relieve perimenopausal symptoms.

Black cohosh is perhaps the best studied of the herbs for menopause, but the studies are contradictory.

On the positive end, there are studies that have shown that black cohosh

- Can effectively reduce the severity, duration, and incidence of hot flashes and night sweats, in some cases by as much as 50 percent
- Reduces problems with sleeping, fatigue, sweating, anxiety, and depression

- Can lower low-density lipoprotein (LDL, "bad" cholesterol) and raise HDL

One randomized, double-blind, placebo-controlled trial (considered to be optimal in research) found that women who took two 2 mg tablets of the popular Remifemin brand of black cohosh twice daily had a fairly dramatic reduction in hot flashes as compared with placebo and conjugated estrogens. The women using black cohosh also had reduced anxiety.

At the same time, there are studies that show no measurable benefit to black cohosh. The highly publicized HALT (Herbal Alternatives for Menopause Trial) study, for example, found that black cohosh used alone or as part of a multiherb treatment did not improve hot flashes and night sweats, and that over a year of evaluation, only prescription hormone therapy resulted in a "clinically important decrease in vasomotor symptoms frequency."

The National Institutes of Health put it, "Although preliminary evidence is encouraging, the currently available data are not sufficient to support a recommendation on the use of black cohosh for menopausal symptoms."

At the same time, because there is some supporting evidence, the World Health Organization has recognized the use of black cohosh for "treatment of climacteric symptoms such as hot flashes, profuse sweating, sleeping disorders and nervous irritability." The North American Menopause Society recommends black cohosh, in conjunction with lifestyle approaches, as a first-line treatment option for women with mild hot flashes and night sweats.

Dr. Tieraona Low Dog believes that black cohosh can be useful, not typically for hot flashes, but for other menopausal symptoms. Says Low Dog:

Black cohosh has traditionally been used for three things: rheumatic pain, melancholy, and sluggish childbirth. So for menopausal women, I've found it more beneficial for joint pain, which is a menopausal symptom for some women, rather than hot flashes. Some of the recent research is suggesting that it is working through the central nervous system and neurotransmitters, which is actually more consistent with its historical use than believing it has "estrogenic properties," which does not appear to be the case. So I often recommend black cohosh for menopausal women who have low-lying depression and body aches, for whom hot flashes are not the main concern.

Occasionally, side effects of black cohosh can include stomach upset, vomiting, dizziness, headaches, visual disturbances, slowed heartbeat, and heaviness in the legs. Some studies have raised significant concerns about the possibility of liver damage with black cohosh. The long-term safety of black cohosh, especially as it affects uterine and breast safety, as well as cancer risk, is not known.

The commercial formulation of black cohosh known as Remifemin has been used in Europe for nearly 50 years, and it appears to be safe according to studies. Remifemin, which contains black cohosh extract equivalent to 20 mg of plant root per tablet, has been studied extensively, and some practitioners suggest that if you are going to use black cohosh, you use this brand specifically. Dr. Jacob Teitelbaum suggests that those who want to try Remifemin start with two tablets twice a day for two months, then drop to one tablet twice a day.

Dr. Risa Kagan advises that patients who want to use black cohosh take certain precautions:

> There is mixed evidence for black cohosh, but if you are taking it, you want to make sure you're getting a good quality, so I'd recommend Remifemin, because it's tested and you know what you're getting. But there is some evidence of liver disease, so we recommend that liver function be checked before and during use of black cohosh.

Other practitioners suggest you avoid staying on black cohosh for extended periods beyond six months to a year. Some experts suggest that women with breast cancer should consider avoiding black cohosh until the effects on breast health have been more thoroughly studied.

DAMIANA

Damiana (*Turnera diffusa* or *Turnera aphrodisiaca*) is an herbal remedy that has mainly been used in the southwestern United States and Mexico. Dr. Tieraona Low Dog highly recommends damiana for menopausal symptoms:

> Damiana is the herb I have used most successfully for menopausal symptoms. Many Latina women would come into my herb shop, asking for damiana. I would ask, "What do you use it for?" and they would tell me that it was helpful for hot flashes and for low sex drive, and generally say, "It makes me feel better."

Dr. Low Dog recommends using damiana in a tea or tincture form. If using the tincture, thirty drops (2 to 3 mL) two or three times a day can work well. For those who take capsules, Dr. Low Dog recommends 500 mg three times a day.

DONG QUAI

Dong quai (*Angelica sinensis*) is a Chinese medicine herb that has been used to treat various gynecological conditions. There are few large-sized trials to establish dong quai's value and effectiveness, but there is some research and evidence suggesting that dong quai root may have some properties to help women in perimenopause/menopause. In particular, as part of combination treatments, it may reduce hot flashes, boost immune function, and improve bone health.

One study looked at a traditional Chinese remedy combining dong quai and chamomile and found that, within a month, there was a significant difference in relief of hot flashes, insomnia, and fatigue in the women taking the remedy, compared with placebo. Other studies have shown that it may be as effective as antianxiety drugs like Valium in helping to relieve stress. There is a suggestion that dong quai stimulates the proliferation of bone cells, which may help protect against osteoporosis.

Note, however, that these studies are all based on customized use of dong quai by Chinese medicine practitioners, and not over-the-counter dong quai supplements. In traditional Chinese medicine, dong quai is never used alone. It is always used in combination with other herbs, and studies of dong quai alone have not shown it to be effective in addressing menopausal symptoms.

Because it does not have an estrogenic effect, it's considered fairly safe. However, there is a possible herb–drug interaction between donq quai and warfarin (the blood-thinning drug Coumadin), so women taking anticoagulants and blood thinners should avoid dong quai.

HERBS FOR SLEEP

For women experiencing sleep problems, there are several herbs that have traditionally been used, including valerian and hops. Valerian (*Valeriana officinalis*) acts as a sedative and may help with insomnia and overall sleep quality. Hops (*Humulus lupulus*) is thought to maintain sleep. Some experts believe that the combination of valerian and hops is optimal in that valerian helps you fall asleep, and hops helps you stay asleep.

A tip: Dr. Jacob Teitelbaum has formulated an herbal sleep remedy for his patients with chronic fatigue and fibromyalgia to help them sleep well without the need for prescription medications. This remedy, End Fatigue Revitalizing Sleep Formula, from PhytoPharmica/Enzymatic Therapies, is now available widely, and it's the one I use and find very helpful. Dr. Teitelbaum combines valerian and hops, along with other ingredients that aid in relaxtion, reducing anxiety, and promoting sleep, including passion flower (*Passiflora incarnata*), L-theanine (an amino acid commonly found in tea), wild lettuce (*Lactuca virosa*), and Jamaica dogwood (*Piscidia piscipula*).

SAGE

Dr. Tieraona Low Dog recommends that women consider a very underused herb, sage, during perimenopause/menopause. Sage's traditional use has been to reduce excessive sweating and relieve night sweats.

According to Dr. Low Dog:

> Sage is an old folk remedy for night sweats and hot flashes, and it can be a useful herb for women in perimenopause/menopause. Many don't like the taste of the tea and prefer capsules. I usually recommend women take 1,000 mg of sage around 4:00 to 6:00 p.m. As an added benefit, it can be good for digestion and the stomach, and may even have some benefits for the brain and memory.

EVENING PRIMROSE OIL

Our bodies need—but cannot make—good fats known as essential fatty acids, so we must get them from the foods we eat or supplements. One essential fatty acid in particular, gamma-linolenic acid (GLA), which is found in evening primrose oil (EPO, *Oenothera biennis* L.), may help reduce inflammation, lessen cramps and PMS symptoms, help with water retention and bloating, and reduce breast pain. It is also known to be helpful in maintaining better moisture balance in skin, hair, and mucous membranes, such as vaginal tissues, eyes, and mouth.

Many practitioners suggest approximately 2,000 mg a day as a level at which benefits might be felt. Studies are inconclusive, but the safety of EPO makes it a supplement that women can consider trying, as results will be felt within several weeks if it is going to work.

EPO typically has few side effects; occasionally, patients complain of mild nausea, diarrhea, gas, and bloating. It should not, however, be used in patients diagnosed with schizophrenia who are taking antipsychotic medication or with anyone taking anticoagulants.

ST. JOHN'S WORT

St. John's wort (*Hypericum perforatum*) has been used for centuries to treat mental disorders, depression, anxiety, sleep disorders, and nerve pain. There is some scientific evidence that it is useful for treating mild to moderate—but not major—depression and mild anxiety.

St. John's wort can have some side effects, including sensitivity to sunlight, dry mouth, dizziness, stomach problems, fatigue, headache, and sexual dysfunction. It can also interact with a number of drugs, including antidepressants, birth control pills, warfarin, and coagulants, as well as with a variety of other heart and immune system medications.

PYCNOGENOL

Pycnogenol (*Pinus pinaster* spp. *atlantica*), a pine bark extract, is a potent antioxidant. For menopausal women, one Scandinavian study found that pycnogenol could help with hot flashes, depression, anxiety, sleep problems, vaginal dryness, fatigue, headache, and lack of sex drive. It is thought to work primarily by improving blood flow. There are no known adverse side effects of pycnogenol, and it's thought that 100 mg, twice a day, is a level that may result in improvement in menopausal symptoms.

VITAMIN E

Vitamin E is widely used for treating hot flashes, but there is limited and mixed research supporting the use. Some studies have shown that use of vitamin E at 800 IU may result in one less hot flash per day. More studies are needed to evaluate the use of vitamin E. But at this level, it's considered safe and may be worth trying.

VITAMIN D

We don't typically think of vitamin D as relating to menopause, except for its role in helping with calcium absorption. But Dr. Jacob Teitelbaum believes that getting some natural vitamin D—"A daily walk in the sunshine!" as he says—is one of the best things we can do to ensure sufficient vitamin D levels. Says Teitelbaum:

> Vitamin D is a critical hormone, not just a vitamin, and it helps support hypothalamic and autonomic function. The hypothalamus helps regulate follicle-stimulating hormone, luteinizing hormone, and estrogen production. So supporting the hypothalamic function, with exercise, sleep—and sunshine (vitamin D)—is critical.

If you are taking vitamin D supplements, many experts recommend approximately 600 IU daily. If you have autoimmune disease or suffer winter seasonal affective disorder or depression, some experts recommend that you supplement with as much as 2,000 IU a day.

CHASTEBERRY/VITEX

Chasteberry (*Vitex agnus-castus*), which is also referred to as vitex, is the berry of a shrub that has been used for centuries to treat various conditions affecting women, including premenstrual problems, breast tenderness, and menstrual irregularities. Some studies suggest that chasteberry works by affecting brain levels of the neurotransmitter dopamine, which then has an impact on the body's prolactin levels. (Prolactin can be a factor in breast tenderness and PMS.) Chasteberry may also help with progesterone balancing.

A number of clinical trials of chasteberry suggest that it can help with the following symptoms:

- Breast pain and tenderness
- Water retention and bloating

- Headache
- Irritability
- Depression
- Fatigue, low energy

Dr. Tieraona Low Dog uses chasteberry for perimenopausal women with irregular cycles, to enhance fertility. In women who are menopausal, Dr. Low Dog uses it primarily for sleep issues and for women who work night shifts who have excessive fatigue.

GINSENG

Panax ginseng has been recommended for menopause complaints. Dr. Tieraona Low Dog has evaluated studies of ginseng and found that, while there is little evidence for any effect on hot flashes, it can help with depression, mood swings, energy, sleep disturbances, and general well-being.

Side effects include headache, upset stomach, and, less commonly, increased blood pressure and raised blood sugar levels.

Complementary Medicine

Several complementary medicine approaches may enhance your overall approach to resolving hormone imbalances: traditional Chinese medicine, osteopathy, adrenal assessment and treatment, and tissue mineral analysis.

TRADITIONAL CHINESE MEDICINE

Physician and Chinese medicine practitioner/acupuncturist Adrienne Clamp, MD, was drawn to the practice of Chinese herbal medicine and acupuncture after an education in conventional medicine.

Things that aren't useful don't last, and while I can share off the top of my head some 50 or 60 drugs that are no longer used just since I've been practicing medicine, many of the Chinese formulas I use have been around for 2,000 years, and are being continuously tweaked. There is longevity and wisdom in Chinese medicine, and I respect the view of looking at people in this holistic way.

Dr. Clamp says, to understand a traditional Chinese medicine view of menopause and thyroid imbalance, you need to consider the concept of "kidney energy." Says Dr. Clamp:

In Chinese medicine, picture a cauldron of water with fire beneath it. The fire below the cauldron is your kidney energy, or yang energy. The water in the cauldron is your yin energy. At menopause, it's as if there is no more water in your cauldron, but the fire continues to burn beneath it. This "false fire"—which is felt by some women as hot flashes—has burned up the water— the "yin energy." Yin is moon—the quiet, nutritive, meditative, soft, more feminine energy. Since we're a yang society—on the go and action-oriented—it's not easy for menopausal women to replenish that "burned up" yin.

During perimenopause, many women are so overtaxed that they don't have enough yin. We are natural multitaskers, raising children, working, cooking dinner, and without hormonal balance, we can become tired or worn out, and get that frazzled feeling like we can't deal. Excitement, stress, and sleep problems all burn away the yin and leave many women yin deficient during perimenopause.

Acupuncture can help to build energy, and herbs can be used to help sustain it.

Dr. Jocelyne Eberstein, a licensed acupuncturist and Chinese medicine practitioner, agrees:

In women in this age group, one of the first areas of decline is with the thyroid and adrenals. What I try to do with Chinese medicine and acupuncture is to help jump-start the hormonal cascade, stimulating it at the level of the pituitary. Then, what you're getting is a downstream cascade of hormonal balance.

Acupuncture requires a trained and licensed practitioner, and Chinese herbal medicine is not a do-it-yourself process, so don't just pick a Chinese herbal formula off the shelf of your health food store. You need a proper Chinese medicine diagnosis and appropriate treatment with acupuncture and herbal remedies, and that can only come from a trained practitioner.

Your health care providers may be a resource for referral to Chinese medicine practitioners and acupuncturists, and some conventional medical practitioners practice acupuncture. In addition, the American Association of Acupuncture and Oriental Medicine (AAAOM) maintains a referral service for licensed practitioners.

TRADITIONAL OSTEOPATHY

An osteopath is a physician trained in the field of osteopathic medicine. Like an MD (medical doctor), a DO (doctor of osteopathic medicine) is a fully trained and licensed physician, and both are considered equal in terms of their authority to diagnose and treat various health conditions, prescribe medications, and perform surgery.

The difference between an MD and a DO is that their educational approach is different. Osteopathic medicine emphasizes the whole person, emphasizing the connection between the musculoskeletal system and disease and symptoms. Both DOs and MDs need an undergraduate degree and four years of medical school. Osteopaths cover the same curriculum as MDs at osteopathic medical schools, plus, an additional 300 to 500 hours of specialized training on the musculoskeletal system. DOs and MDs then typically do two to six years of internship and residency programs, pass state licensing exams, and obtain continuing education to remain certified. Like MDs, DOs can specialize in particular areas of medicine.

Some osteopaths take a hands-on osteopathic approach, using cranial and musculoskeletal systems to help restore balance and relieve neurologic, respiratory, digestive, and other symptoms. Osteopaths who practice using only the hands-on treatments tend to refer to themselves as "traditional" osteopaths.

Scott Kwiatkowski, DO, a traditional osteopath practicing in Silver Spring, Maryland, believes that osteopathy can be an excellent part of an integrative approach to hormonal imbalance. Says Kwiatkowski:

I like to view the body as a house, with frame, plumbing, and electricity. The bones are the frame. The circulatory and lymph systems are the plumbing. And the brain, spinal column, and nerves are the electrical system. Osteopaths work with the frame—the structure—to improve the circulatory and electrical systems—meaning we work with the bones, to help improve the health of the circulatory, lymph, nervous system, and hormones.

In dealing with a woman who is going through perimenopause, osteopathically, I look at her as a whole person. Using the tenets of osteopathy, people have all they need contained within them, and the body knows how to regulate itself. It's a self-healing machine. So I look at structure—how is the body looking, hormonally, with evaluation of sex hormones, adrenals, and the thyroid—and work to rebalance.

In my own case, I have regularly turned to osteopathic treatment, and it's an important part of my own integrative approach to hormone balance and wellness.

While many osteopaths work as general practitioners and incorporate some hands-on work into their regular practice, you might find that the approach of a "traditional" osteopath to be a wonderful additional to your wellness approach. Appendix A has several referral sources for osteopathic physicians.

Assess the Adrenals

When there is evidence of thyroid dysfunction, it's important to also consider evaluating adrenal function. The adrenal glands, part of the endocrine system and located on top of the kidneys, coordinate the body's response to stress, both long-term regular stress and the short-term, "fight or flight" stressors. To deal with more chronic stress, the adrenal glands release cortisol, the body's "steroid" hormone. To cope with urgent stress, the body releases adrenaline.

Both releases have metabolic effects on the body.

In many women, by our forties, we are dealing with suboptimal adrenal function and adrenal imbalances. Women may have low adrenals in the morning, with levels that become too high later in the day, which is not a normal pattern. Or, in some cases, levels are consistently too low—evidence of underactive adrenal function.

Dr. Adrienne Clamp incorporates adrenal analysis into her overall hormone-balancing approach. According to Clamp:

> The role of suboptimal adrenal function is not very well addressed or recognized. It can wreak havoc and undermine health and wellness if not addressed. When thyroid function appears to be normal and still someone suffers with all the symptoms of hypothyroidism, often adrenal hypofunction is to blame. Diagnosis can be suggested by the history of recent or prolonged stress, or recurrent bouts of serious illness. It is best confirmed by measurement of saliva cortisol levels throughout the day and evening. Measurement of the other hormones made by the adrenal gland such as DHEA [dehydroepiandrosterone] sulfate and aldosterone is also helpful.
>
> Treatment of the adrenal gland dysfunction depends on the pattern. I usually turn to herbal adaptogens first, as well as recommending work on stress reduction by means such as meditation, relaxation, learning different coping mechanisms, and psychological counseling, among others. Sometimes hormone

replacement is needed and in extreme cases of hypofunction, even low doses of cortisol, though this is typically only after trying the other approaches.

Assess Mineral Imbalances

Holistic nutritionist Dr. Ann Louise Gittleman believes that one of the most important things women with hormonal imbalances can do is to have their minerals evaluated for deficiencies, excesses, or imbalances. According to Gittleman:

> The adrenal glands act as a backup system for the ovaries, and when the adrenals weaken and the metabolism slows, copper tends to accumulate. When we're under stress, we can also develop a zinc deficiency, which can then lead to adrenal insufficiency, which then leads to copper excess or a copper/zinc imbalance. In perimenopause, progesterone deficiency or an estrogen-dominance estrogen/progesterone balance can also cause copper to accumulate. And when we see that imbalance, we also frequently see an underactive thyroid.

Dr. Gittleman recommends that women facing thyroid or reproductive hormone imbalances have what's known as a tissue mineral analysis, to evaluate the levels of minerals and pinpoint deficiencies, excesses, or imbalances. The tissue mineral analysis, which is done with a hair sample, evaluates the levels of exposure to a host of minerals and toxins. According to Dr. Gittleman:

> My feeling is that it's a key to how women can better go through menopause. Copper imbalance is the most prevalent imbalance I find. Copper overload also causes a sluggish liver, and you can't metabolize toxins or hormones, so you can become bloated and hormone deficient.

I had my tissue mineral analysis done, and we found some interesting imbalances, as well as some toxic exposures, including slightly high mercury exposure, which is often associated with hypothyroidism. I'm now working to balance these issues nutritionally. But this test found a number of issues, and the test results included a great deal of information about what I can do to help address the imbalances and problems.

If you're interested in a tissue mineral analysis, some holistic doctors can do this and interpret the results. Appendix A includes information on how you can order your own tissue mineral analysis testing and where to get results interpreted.

chapter 7

Transforming
YOUR DIET

One cannot think well, love well, sleep well, if one has not dined well.

—*Virginia Woolf*

Many of the practitioners who shared their advice for this book emphasized how critical it is that we make good nutrition and a healthy diet a core of our overall health focus in perimenopause/menopause. There are a number of reasons to pay particular attention to diet during this time of life. First, many women gain weight during the transition from perimenopause to menopause. If there is a thyroid slowdown taking place at the same time, the metabolism is suffering a double whammy. So not only is eating well important for your overall health and hormonal balance, it's also critical to prevent weight gain due to slowed metabolism and hormonal shifts. Ob-gyn Dr. Risa Kagan shares her thoughts on why it's so important to adapt your diet:

> Diet modification is essential. . . . You need to be looking at what you're eating and how you're eating. Not gaining those extra ten

pounds during the forty-five to fifty-five age range is going to help you later in life, in terms of maintaining a normal body weight and reducing joint pain. You have to find what is going to work for you, and it has to be a way of life.

Second, improved nutrition can help with specific symptoms of perimenopause/menopause, such as hot flashes. Holistic physician Dr. Martin Mulders says that "while changing the diet is the hardest thing to do, changing the diet is perhaps one of the most important things that women can do to help with their hormone-related symptoms." He shares the story of one patient:

A woman came in in menopause—she was having twenty hot flashes a day, she was on Premarin and Provera, and she was seeing me as a "last resort." She also had digestive problems. I put her on a gluten-free, dairy-free diet. Three weeks later, she came back, and instead of twenty hot flashes, she was having only two or three hot flashes a day, she had lost ten pounds, and her digestive problems were gone.

Third, many thyroid patients have less-than-optimal immune systems (especially the many millions of us with autoimmune Hashimoto's disease). Dr. Mulders says that we can view the immune system like a big bucket. When the bucket runs over, we call it a "disease." When you take junk out of the diet, you're essentially "scraping out the bucket" and leaving more space. When you add proper nutrients and support the hormones, "you actually make the bucket bigger."

Finally, heart health becomes a concern at this time, as heart disease becomes more prevalent in women over age fifty. So improving our diet is even more essential as we get older. (Don't forget that thyroid problems typically increase our risk for heart disease somewhat, even more reason to make sure your diet is heart healthy.)

There is no specific "menopause diet" that is a perfect fit for every woman. But there are a number of practical and effective recommendations that can help you feel and live well and apply, across the board, to most women who are dealing with hormonal changes due to thyroid problems, perimenopause, or menopause.

Chew, Chew, Chew

I love this recommendation, and I think it's a wonderful one to start with. It comes from New York City–based holistic nutrition counselor Irma Jennings, who spoke with me at length for this chapter. Irma works with many women who are experiencing hormonal fluctuations, to help improve diet and nutrition. She believes that one of the most fundamental changes that women can make with regard to what we eat is to chew. In her presentations, Irma hands out raisins and has women eat one raisin, eyes closed, chewing it as many as twenty times, to experience the sensation of thoroughly chewing, savoring the flavor, and observing how chewing releases digestive enzymes and allows them to work properly. Says Irma:

> Chewing is such an important action that is often rushed through using our fork as a shovel, and is often sandwiched between our multitasking, such as watching TV, reading, checking e-mail, working, talking on the cell phone, and dealing with children or any other interruptions. Gulping our food bypasses the enjoyment of feeding ourselves on the deepest level. The digestion process actually begins in the mouth, where we digest carbohydrates, simple and complex, and veggies, fruits, grains, etc., with the release of the enzyme in the saliva known as amylase. The more we chew, five to ten times, the easier the digestive process will be.

Reduce Portion Sizes

Americans eat huge portions. Even if you're focusing on healthy foods, large portions can derail your efforts at good nutrition or weight management. To help reduce portions, use a smaller plate for your meals, and start with a small portion (and wait ten minutes before taking seconds). At most restaurants, where portions tend to be especially large, make it a habit to ask for a takeaway container or doggie bag at the beginning of the meal, and put some of your meal aside to eat at another time.

Eat More Fruits and Vegetables

It sounds so basic, but a healthy diet should include a good supply of fruits and vegetables. If you are trying to lose weight or are struggling with a slower metabolism, emphasize vegetables over fruit. Limit the higher glycemic fruits like bananas and starchy vegetables like potatoes and instead choose nutrition-rich, low-calorie green vegetables and high-fiber fruits like berries and apples.

You can limit high-glyemic carbohydrates while still eating a vegetable- and fruit-rich diet. *The South Beach Diet* and its updated edition, *The South Beach Diet Supercharged,* for example, have excellent recommendations on a nutritional approach that is well suited for people with thyroid problems who are in hormonal flux and who want to eat well and either maintain or lose weight.

Since fruits and vegetables are so good, should you become a vegetarian? Dr. Annemarie Colbin, a nutritionist, author, and founder of the Natural Gourmet Institute, a prestigious cooking school in New York City, says not necessarily. Dr. Colbin ate a vegetarian diet and followed macrobiotic diets at various points in her life, but she said that at menopause, she craved red meat and did not deny herself. Says Colbin:

> Vegetarianism really only works for those who do it without thinking. It feels natural to some people; they just don't even have to think about it. If you have to really work at being a vegetarian, then it's not for you.

For those who are vegetarians, Dr. Colbin cautions against being what she refers to as a "junk food vegetarian."

Junk food vegetarians often live on sugar, sweets, and canned foods, which have nothing to do with health.

Eat Healthier, Low-Fat Sources of Protein

Everyone can focus on shifting from high-fat protein sources like red meat, toward more of the healthy, low-fat sources of protein in your diet, including nuts, seeds, and legumes (like beans). If you are a meat eater, you don't need to stop eating meat, but you should cut back on the amount of meat you eat. When you do eat meat or poultry, use organic, hormone-free, grass-fed meat and poultry whenever possible, and trim visible fat. And try to choose the lower fat cuts of meat, including

- Ground beef with less than 10 percent fat
- Filet mignon
- Top loin
- Sirloin
- Top and bottom round and round steak
- Rump roast
- Flank steak
- London broil
- Pork loin and tenderloin

With poultry, skinless white meat is always your best choice.

Eliminate Processed Foods and Refined Sugars

Most of the practitioners I spoke with felt that eliminating processed foods and refined sugars as much as possible is an important nutritional goal for women.

Nutritionist Irma Jennings summarized some of the concerns:

Processed foods typically have a long shelf life due to the preservatives and processed added oils. They often come in brightly colored packaging to attract the attention of the consumer and are typically high in sugars, such as high fructose corn syrup and artificial sweeteners.

Sugar can easily become an addiction. As with any addiction, the body leads one to believe that sugar is needed. The packaged/fast food industry relies on this addiction to sell their foods.

Sugars are acid forming and known for leaching calcium from our bones. The preponderance of sugar in most processed and packaged foods (even in many so-called health foods) and in our American culture hides the fact that refined sugar is a recent, and growing, phenomenon.

The processed and sugar-laden packaged foods are most often found in the center aisles of the average supermarket, so many nutrition experts suggest you shop the perimeter of the grocery store, where the fruits and vegetables are typically located.

Ignore the claims on processed and packaged foods that promise "low-fat," "low-carb," "low sugar," or "fortified with" because these are typically misleading.

Eat Organic, Pesticide-Free, Hormone-Free Food

Irma Jennings recommends buying organic foods whenever possible:

Whole organic produce is far superior. They are grown in healthy soils, whose crops are rotated from year to year, allowing the soil to retain its nutrients, as opposed to the depleted, over-farmed produce that we find at the markets. They naturally have a significant nutritional impact, are rich in the vitamins, minerals, and phytonutrients our body needs, and are grown without synthetic pesticides, herbicides, chemical fertilizers, or hormones.

Incorporate Good Fats

If you are trying to lose weight, you may need to cut back on fats in general, because they tend to be higher in calories, compared with protein and carbohydrates. But eating healthy in the perimenopausal/menopausal years does not necessarily mean eating low-fat; it means eating some good fat. As discussed in Chapter 3, cholesterol, which is a component of fat, is the building block for all our sex hormones. Dr. Annemarie Colbin explains:

> I don't like low-fat diets; we need good fats, for fat-soluble vitamins, for hormones, for the brain and the nervous system, and to feel that we've had enough to eat. But fats should be good quality—organic butter, extra virgin olive oil, coconut oil. You need to include some fat in the diet; otherwise you're not going to be happy.

So minimize or eliminate the saturated and trans fats, found in red meat, full-fat dairy products, many fried foods, and many processed foods. Instead, focus on polyunsaturated and monounsaturated fats found, for example, in nuts, oily fish, avocado, olive oil, canola oil, and flaxseed oil.

About Drinks: Water, Coffee, Soda, and Alcohol

First, remember not to drink your calories. Sugary soft drinks, juices, and special coffee drinks are all calorie-laden. Studies have shown that beverages do not fill you up like foods, and even if you drink these high-calorie beverages, you'll still eat the same amount.

Nutritionist Irma Jennings suggests that we should replace sodas in particular with other drinks. According to Jennings:

> Soft drinks are high in phosphoric acid and sugar, making these drinks high acidic. Calcium is the main mineral the body uses to neutralize that acid. Phosphoric acid depletes calcium levels by causing it to be pulled from the bones. In my research on bone health, I have never come across one article that suggests that diet soda is good for bone health. If you drink diet soda, start adding one glass of water a day for a week. Then replace one diet soda with a glass of water.

Jennings also encourages women to drink plenty of clean water. But how much water should we be getting? Recommendations vary, but acupuncturist and holistic practitioner Dr. Jocelyne Eberstein feels that perimenopausal and menopausal women should be drinking at least 100 ounces of clean water a day.

How and where you get your clean water will depend on how much effort and money you want to put into your water supply. Some women use a Brita, PUR, or similar filter to remove basic impurities from tap water. Others buy calcium-rich mineral waters, like Perrier and San Pellegrino, for regular drinking or have a water service that delivers spring water to the home or office. Some households install more elaborate, higher-end reverse osmosis and specialized whole-house water filter systems to remove toxins.

As far as alcohol is concerned, we know that the jury is out on how healthy it is. Some studies show that moderate drinking, that is, less than two glasses of wine a day, may help heart health. But more than two drinks a day may increase breast cancer risk. If you like to have a drink, be moderate, and keep in mind that the calories in alcohol can add up. For example, a regular beer has 150 calories in a 12-ounce serving, most spirits have 60 to 70 calories in a 1-ounce serving, wines range from 80 to 10 calories a glass, and margaritas and other sweet drinks can have 200 or more calories per glass.

If you are having night sweats, consider eliminating alcohol entirely. Tucson, Arizona–based holistic physician Molly Roberts has found that, for her patients who are experiencing night sweats, eliminating all alcohol frequently lessens the frequency and severity of night sweats or eliminates them completely.

Go Japanese

Nutritionist Dr. Annemarie Colbin believes that it's not as much the soy, but rather the seaweed and fish in the Japanese diet, that may play a role in minimizing menopausal symptoms for Japanese women. There's the additional benefit of these foods helping thyroid function, due to their natural iodine content.

Dr. Colbin recommends we eat incorporate more Japanese-style cooking, and, as Colbin told me, "eat a Japanese meal twice a week—some sushi, miso soup, and seaweed salad."

As a sushi lover myself, I have no problem incorporating this recommendation into my diet. If you don't have time to go to a Japanese restaurant or can't cook Japanese-style meals, Dr. Colbin recommends you add a bit of nori to your diet. Nori is a dried seaweed that comes in thin sheets; according to Dr. Colbin, you can add it to soup or even eat it plain as a snack.

(Note: Dr. Colbin has a wonderful video, *The Basics of Healthy Cooking*, that in less than two hours teaches you about healthy cooking, even how to roll sushi. I highly recommend it if you want to try incorporating Japanese cooking at home.)

Eat More High-Fiber Foods

Aim to get 25 to 30 grams of fiber every day, ideally from foods. High-fiber foods include bran cereals like All-Bran, Bran Buds, 100% Bran, and Raisin Bran, whole grain breads, lentils, lima beans and other beans, and most nuts.

High-fiber vegetables:

- Beans
- Broccoli*
- Brussels sprouts*
- Cabbage*
- Carrots
- Chickpeas/garbanzo beans
- Eggplant
- Greens: collards, kale, turnip greens*
- Lima beans
- Mushrooms
- Spinach*
- Sweet potatoes

*These high-fiber vegetables are also goitrogenic, meaning that they promote thyroid enlargement and can potentially cause or aggravate hypothyroidism. Typically, the risk is highest when these foods are consumed raw, regularly, and in substantial quantity. Cooking eliminates most goitrogenic properties.

High-fiber fruits:

- Apples
- Avocado
- Bananas
- Berries: blueberies, blackberries, raspberries, and so on
- Dried fruits: figs, raisins, apricots, dates, and so on

Note: While they are rich in fiber and nutrients, avocados and dried fruits are not low-calorie foods.

Remember that if you are taking thyroid medication, fiber-rich foods can interfere with the effective absorption of your thyroid medication. So if you start a high-fiber diet, you should have your thyroid rechecked eight to twelve weeks after making this change, to assess whether you need a dosage readjustment.

Calcium (and Calcium-rich Foods)

Many experts recommend that after menopause, a woman should be getting at least 1,500 mg of calcium daily, to help prevent loss of bone mineral density. Perimenopausal women should be getting 1,000 to 1,200 mg of calcium daily. Ideally, calcium should be obtained from food. The following are some guidelines to calcium content:

- Milk, regular or skim, 1 cup: 300 mg
- Calcium-fortified orange juice, 1 cup: 300 mg
- Yogurt, regular or fat-free, 1 cup: 400 mg
- Cheddar cheese, 1 ounce: about 200 mg
- Salmon, 3 ounces: 200 mg

Other foods high in calcium are

- Various greens, such as collards, broccoli, kale, and spinach (remember to cook them to remove their goitrogenic potential to slow down your thyroid and contribute to hypothyroidism)
- Sea vegetables such as wakame, kombu, and dulse (don't forget that some thyroid patients are sensitive to iodine, and overconsumption of these iodine-rich vegetables may trigger or aggravate thyroid conditions)
- Mineral waters, including Perrier and San Pellegrino

It can be hard to eat enough calcium-rich foods to get sufficient amounts of calcium, so many women need supplements. You can use something as simple and inexpensive as calcium carbonate (for example, Tums) or calcium citrate supplements. Many practitioners suggest you avoid calcium products made from bone meal, dolomite, or oyster shells, as these products may contain unnecessary lead.

Since you can't absorb more than around 500 mg of calcium, spread out calcium supplementation throughout the day. It's best absorbed when taken with food.

Important note: If you are taking Synthroid, Armour, or any other thyroid hormone replacement drug, calcium supplements and calcium-fortified products can interfere with absorption of these drugs, so allow at least four hours between taking your thyroid hormone drug and calcium-rich foods or supplements.

Watch Goitrogens and Soy

While making sure we get more vegetables in the diet can be healthy, we also need to be careful about the effect these foods can have on the thyroid when consumed improperly or in too large a quantity.

Goitrogens are chemicals found in certain foods that promote formation of goiters and can slow down the thyroid, causing hypothyroidism. Specifically, goitrogens inhibit the body's ability to use iodine, blocking the process by which iodine becomes the thyroid hormones thyroxine (T4) and triiodothyronine (T3).

If you don't have a thyroid gland due to surgery, or if you've had radioactive iodine treatment, you don't have to be particularly concerned about goitrogens. If you still have a functional thyroid, however, you need to be more concerned and careful not to eat goitrogens uncooked in large quantities. The enzymes involved in the formation of goitrogenic materials in plants can be partially destroyed by cooking. Eating moderate amounts of goitrogenic foods, raw or cooked, is usually not a problem for most women.

A list of common and potent goitrogens is featured in Chapter 2.

Soy, in addition to being a goitrogen, is a plant estrogen—or phytoestrogen—which means that soy can act as a weak hormone, operating like estrogen in the body. I've discussed soy at greater length in Chapter 6.

chapter 8

EXERCISE

I have to exercise in the morning before
my brain figures out what I'm doing.

—*Marsha Doble*

In the course of writing this book, I interviewed dozens of practitioners—doctors, naturopaths, holistic health practitioners, and hormone researchers—and almost every single expert said that there is one important thing that women can do to feel and look better through perimenopause and beyond: move our bodies.

It may sound simplistic, but there is a great deal of evidence that physical exercise—that includes everything from basic movement to walking to yoga—can help with both the physical and mental symptoms associated with hormonal changes.

Dr. Jocelyne Eberstein emphasizes that it's important that we move the body every day,

even if just a few minutes a day. Everybody has fifteen minutes for a walk, just to get the lungs moving, your breathing going, and allow your nervous system to discharge. Then there's a coherence in the body.

Gynecologist and menopause expert Risa Kagan, MD, says that women between forty-five and fifty-five often exercise less and eat in a different way, due to lifestyle, aging, kids, career, and so on.

It gets harder and harder as you get older, so women need to move. Exercise is essential for feeling good, for bone strength, and for balance. We need some form of exercise every day.

Besides generally improving quality of life, research has shown that exercise can benefit perimenopausal/menopausal/hypothyroid women in a number of specific ways:

- Reduced number, intensity, or duration of hot flashes and night sweats
- Improved mood
- Less depression
- Reduced anxiety
- Better sex drive
- Better sleep
- More energy, less fatigue
- Weight control, less weight gain
- Help in redistributing weight that is shifting due to hormones
- Fewer body aches
- Better bone density
- Better heart health

Ob-gyn and hormone expert Dr. Jan Shifren says that exercise is one of the most important things that women can do. "It's clear: women who exercise are physically and psychologically healthier," she says. In studies that compared exercise and hormone therapy for menopausal symptoms, while the symptoms were reduced by both approaches, the quality of life was improved only for women who exercised.

If you are athletic and already have an exercise program in place, then you've already laid the foundation for a healthier, happier hormonal change. Whatever exercise you're doing, make sure that it is meeting three key criteria:

- Are you getting enough exercise?
- Does your exercise program build muscle?
- Does your exercise program improve lymphatic function?

Let's take a look at these key issues.

First, as far as the amount of exercise is concerned, you probably need more exercise than you think. Keep in mind that experts are now saying that to maintain weight, we need 150 minutes of exercise per week, but to lose weight, we need an estimated 275 minutes each week. That's four and a half hours each week, optimally spread out over five or more days.

Second, in terms of building muscle, with metabolism slowing each year during perimenopause and beyond (and an underactive thyroid slowing the metabolism even further), a key to preventing weight gain is muscle-building exercise. Muscle is metabolically active, a fancy way of saying that muscle burns more calories than fat. So let's say you compared two friends, both of them 150-pound women. If one of these women has 20 percent body fat, and the other has 28 percent body fat, compared with her friend, the woman with less fat can actually eat more calories without gaining weight. (Or, if they are trying to lose weight, the woman with less fat and more muscle won't need to cut quite as many calories, or exercise as much as her friend, to achieve weight loss.)

Third, exercise should help improve lymphatic function. Your lymphatic system's purpose is to absorb excess fluid, fat, toxins, and waste products, filter them out, and return the filtered liquid (known as lymph) to the bloodstream. The body's lymph vessels— which are like blood vessels in a way—are found throughout the body. So, in many ways, the lymphatic system is like the circulatory system, but with one key difference. The circulatory system has a pump—the heart—to move fluid. The lymphatic system has no pump; the only way lymph fluid is moved through its vessels is through movement, massage, and deep breathing. Some of the best ways to move lymph are activities that involve muscle contraction and deep breathing, including skipping, running, trampolining, re-bounding (on a mini trampoline), and an exercise approach known as T-Tapp that I'll discuss a bit later in this chapter.

According to naturopathic doctor, nutritionist, and weight loss expert Ann Louise Gittleman, proper lymphatic function is critical, because if the liver can be viewed as the body's filter, lymph channels are the body's drainage system. Says Gittleman:

> The lymphatic system needs a better press agent, because, despite its crucial importance, many women aren't aware of it. Healthy lymph is pumped, and what pumps the lymph is exercise. This is one way that we know nature intended us to be active, because the lymphatic system only works when we are moving. It's not involuntary, like our heart pumping blood. But Mother Nature didn't count on eighty-hour work weeks and sedentary jobs at desks.

When we don't move, the lymphatic system is unable to operate, and it can get clogged, backed up, and sluggish. This, says Gittleman, causes us to bloat and swell; tissues can become waterlogged, even adding as much as five to fifteen pounds of extra water weight that is hard to shed. It can also make your immune system less effective and worsen fatigue. According to Gittleman, poor lymphatic function also translates into poor absorption, because if tissues are already full of liquid, they are unable to properly absorb nutrients.

Besides a lack of movement, other things that can negatively affect lymphatic function are poor posture, tight clothes, and sitting for long periods.

Choosing Your Exercise

The type of exercise or physical activity you get is less important than making sure you build it into your life on a regular basis. And that, for many of us who are not athletic or naturally drawn to exercise, is the challenge. Some of the things that can help you make exercise a regular part of your life:

- Exercise with a friend.
- Join a gym or health club.
- Exercise earlier in the day.
- Schedule your exercise on your calendar or personal digital assistant (PDA).
- Take advantage of gyms at your workplace: schedule early morning, lunch, or after-work workouts.
- Free up time by watching one less TV program, and use that time for exercise.
- Entertain yourself: listen to audiobooks or watch TV or movies while exercising. (Some people even tell themselves they can only listen/watch when they're working out.)
- Sneak activity into your day: park farther away, take the stairs, go for a walk at lunch, do housework and yard work, play with children, get a dog, clean vigorously.
- Don't use thyroid problems as an excuse not to exercise, unless your doctor has told you specifically that you can't.

As for exercise, the key is consistency. You have to find something that you love and that works well for you, and stick to it. Holistic nutritionist Irma Jennings has some thoughts:

Finding the exercise program that best fits your personality is key. Personally, I am not attracted to the gym, but I use it on days of inclement weather. I love fast walking outside along the river with small hand weights. Many of my clients enjoy yoga, qi gong, Nia movement, belly dancing, dancing, swimming, water aerobics, and bike riding. Daily movement keeps the body alive, the joints lubricated, and the mind active.

If you're not the least bit interested in an "exercise program," then take the advice of Jacob Teitelbaum, MD, an expert on thyroid disease, metabolism, and chronic fatigue syndrome. Says Dr. Teitelbaum, "Just go outside, get sunshine, and get walking."

According to Teitelbaum:

Walking as exercise helps support hypothalamic and autonomic function, which can help to balance sex hormones, reduce hot flashes, and improve sleep quality. And walking outdoors raises vitamin D levels. Vitamin D is not only a vitamin, but a critical hormone that is essential for immune function.

Dr. Jan Shifren agrees:

You don't need to go to the gym, and you don't need expensive equipment. Really, you can get out and walk a half hour a day. Add music or a friend to walk with, and you get an even better boost of well-being.

Walking is inexpensive and requires no special equipment besides a decent pair of walking shoes. Even beginners can start. We've all heard the success stories of people who start out walking around the block, then gradually increase the distance until they're walking miles each day or even running a marathon.

If you're just getting into walking for fitness, you might want to follow a simple walking schedule, with five walking sessions each week, as follows:

- **Week 1**: start with fifteen-minute walks that include five minutes of slow walking, five minutes of brisker walking, and five minutes of slow walking.

- **Week 2**: add two minutes of brisk walking in the middle, for a total of seventeen minutes of walking.

- **Week 3**: add two minutes of brisk walking in the middle, for a total of nineteen minutes of walking.

- **By adding only two minutes a week, you'll be taking forty-minute power walks after only twelve weeks.**

Music may help you keep a good pace. With an iPod, MP3 player, or portable CD player, you can listen to your own customized playlists of energizing music. You may even want to try an audio walking program. Fitness expert Joanie Greggains has a terrific one-hour walking program called *Pacewalk*, which is available on a CD or by download from the Internet. With Joanie's CD, after a warm-up segment, the music sets the pace, and you follow the beat for ten minutes, twenty minutes, sixty minutes or longer, based on your fitness level. A number of other audio walking programs, featuring different styles of music, are available by CD or download.

A great way to balance out walking is to add yoga. Yoga has been found to be helpful to perimenopausal women and to thyroid patients. Even eight weeks of regular yoga practice was found in some studies to reduce hot flashes, stress, and anxiety in women.

Certain yoga poses, known as inversion poses, can be especially helpful. Says holistic practitioner Dr. Jocelyne Eberstein: "I recommend inversion poses, because they give blood to the thyroid area to help regenerate the thyroid. Inversion poses also help increase serotonin and aid in digestion."

You don't have to be a yogi doing headstands, however. "Even propping your legs up on the wall is enough," says Eberstein.

My Favorite Exercise Program: T-Tapp

I'll be honest: I'm not the least bit athletic, and I have little skill when it comes to exercise. But as a writer, I'm chained to my desk too many hours a day, my back frequently gets creaky and stiff, and as a thyroid patient, my metabolism isn't optimal, so I absolutely need to exercise. For about four years straight, I had been doing Pilates—not especially well but regularly—thanks to a trainer who came to my home and worked out with my best friend and me. For me, the convenience of having the trainer at my house, plus the social incentive of working out with my friend—and the fun of a meal and chatting afterwards—was the motivation I needed to stay with the program. Pilates helped my energy a bit and kept my legs and arms toned, but the main physical benefit was that it kept me flexible and free of back pain. It didn't really do much in terms of slimming or changing my body shape. But my trainer moved away, my friend started exercising with her husband, and I was cast adrift, in search of a new exercise program.

This was not an easy prospect. There was a hilarious attempt at dance aerobics. (I'm one of those utterly uncoordinated people who trip over their own feet when the instructor calls "Grapevine! Grapevine!") And you don't even want to hear about my experiences with step aerobics and "hot" yoga.

So when I kept getting e-mails from readers telling me about T-Tapp, I was interested. The readers were sharing their stories about being hypothyroid and trying to lose weight and tone up. Nothing had been working until they started doing this program called T-Tapp. (Seriously, when I first head the name, I thought it must be some sort of tap dancing exercise program.)

One reader, Denise, wrote:

> I have been diagnosed as hypothyroid for a number of years, but
> have never felt normal and have continued to gain weight until I

don't know who that is in the mirror. Over the last three months I have worked out an hour a day, T-Tapping. It is a fabulous workout. I forced myself to do it because I had become nothing but flab and had no energy. I was desperate to find a way to build some muscle, hoping it would help to reduce the fat. In three months, I have actually lost ten inches. The T-Tapp team is great and very encouraging. I was told to do the routine less often for a better result (!), and it works. Amazing!

After receiving a number of similar e-mails, I decided I had to find out more. I learned that T-Tapp was created by exercise physiologist and rehabilitative fitness specialist Teresa Tapp; hence the name. There was no tap dancing at all; instead, T-Tapp was a series of unique movements designed to improve spinal alignment, flexibility, and strength, as well as to build muscle, improve lymphatic function, raise metabolism, and control glucose levels. Plus, T-Tapp had a built-in focus on rehabilitation. You didn't need to be an athlete to get started. The program promised results.

In my own case, the first week I T-Tapped, I did the routine, which is easy to follow, three times, about forty minutes each session. I lost twelve inches in that first week alone, with three inches of it at my waist. It wasn't hard to convince me to keep T-Tapping. (Needless to say, after that first week's loss, I'm not losing twelve inches a week, but as long as I do my T-Tapp workout several times a week, I'm making progress.) Meanwhile, everything is firming up, I wake up without aches and pains, and my body is far more flexible. Going up and down the stairs, my legs feel lighter, stronger.

I didn't understand how even a week of T-Tapp, compared with months of Pilates, could have such an immediate effect on my body in terms of inches lost. Teresa Tapp explained it:

While T-Tapp has some elements similar to Pilates and even yoga, I specifically designed the sequence of exercises in T-Tapp to provide a comprehensively nonimpact, aerobic conditioning workout that activates muscles at various points, for maximum effectiveness. But with T-Tapp, your muscles don't bulk up. My approach helps you develop longer, leaner, denser muscles, and these muscles act like girdles to support and cinch in key areas.

An additional benefit of T-Tapp is that Teresa Tapp designed it to specifically optimize lymphatic function. According to Tapp, T-Tapp is not only isotonic (like most exercise) and neurokinetic, or communicating mind to muscle (like Pilates and yoga), but

with T-Tapp I add leverage isometrics. These are acupressure points to intensify the mind-to-muscle nerve transmission, which optimizes isometric activation. Using small added components—even something as simple as changing the position of your thumb, or keeping your knee to your little toe—activates muscles better than if you are just thinking about it.

T-Tapp features a variety of workouts, including exercises you can do lying on the floor, seated in a chair, using a broom for balance, and walking, as well as a number of routines and approaches. I particularly like the availability of the T-Tapp More program, which is, as Tapp describes it, for people with more to lose, more physical limitations/injuries/health issues, or more candles on the cake. If you haven't been working out regularly, T-Tapp More is a wonderful way to ease into exercising and enjoy results. And you don't end up flat on your back for two days, exhausted, after doing a workout.

If you don't have an exercise program that you regularly follow, I would encourage you to find out more about T-Tapp and adopt it as your program. Even if you participate in regular exercise, adding T-Tapp to your exercise regimen can help improve your overall fitness and the results you get from your workouts.

Mindful Movement for Menopause Management by T-Tapp

For several decades, Teresa Tapp has worked with perimenopausal and menopause patients, as well as women with a slowed metabolism due to thyroid problems, so she knows what works for us. I was thrilled when Teresa offered to develop the following special sequence of T-Tapp exercises to help us with hormonal balancing, blood sugar management, and toning of key areas.

In addition to this wonderful program Teresa Tapp has created and I've featured here in the book, Teresa has developed a companion instructional DVD on *Mindful Movement for Menopause Management*. To find out more about the menopause DVD, Teresa's best-selling book, *Fit and Fabulous in 15 Minutes*, and all the helpful T-Tapp exercise DVDs and products, see Appendix A and my Web site, www.menopausethyroid.com, or visit www.t-tapp.com.

A SPECIAL MESSAGE FROM TERESA TAPP: "YES, YOU CAN!"

Have you ever heard the saying "When you put your mind to it, anything is possible?" It's true! In fact, that's one of the reasons I say and think, *Yes, You Can* all the time.

Yes, You Can has always been my mantra, not only to deliver positive energy and endurance, but to help others improve their mental focus and create mindful movement. I believe optimizing mind-to-muscle transmission is one of the primary reasons why T-Tapp workouts help women rebuild metabolic function, improve hormonal balance, and sleep better. Using mindful movement during regular activity can also help your body burn more calories and control blood sugar throughout the day.

Along with burning calories and fat, the following sequence of mindful movement is designed to help your body improve mental clarity, lymphatic function, and lessen inflammation too. Sequence is important so your body can progressively develop strength and flexibility, as well as provide protection and spinal support. Each exercise works five to seven muscles, from origin to insertion, layer by layer, to cinch in your frame. This is why T-Tappers can target trim areas of concern and report dramatic inch loss.

Application of form is very important, so read all the instructions and study the photos before trying each exercise. You should feel heat radiate through your spine and all through your body as you progressively warm up. Best of all, the more neurokinetically connected your body becomes (mind to muscle), the faster you will feel this, even to the back of your hands and tops of your feet. Neurokinetic transmission is the foundation of mindful movement that empowers your muscles to increase intensity without increasing repetitions or using equipment.

Last, always perform each exercise to your best ability so you can achieve optimal results. Understanding how to move your body to maximize physiological function, in addition to calorie expenditure, is the secret to looking and feeling better. Remember, it's not what you do but how you do it!

SOME DEFINITIONS

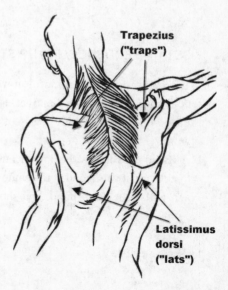

Trapezius ("traps")

Latissimus dorsi ("lats")

KLT — knees to little toe, a key T-Tapp position that involves pushing your knees out toward your little toes
Lats — the latissimus dorsi muscles, the large, flat muscles on the trunk, posterior to the arm, and partly covered by the trapezius muscles ("traps")
Traps — the trapezius muscles

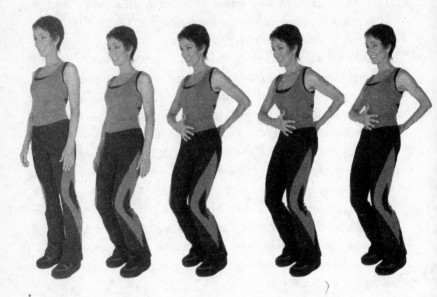

Photo 1

Step 1
SET-UP SEQUENCE/T-TAPP STANCE

The ability to create mindful movement starts by putting your body into alignment and activating internal muscles with the T-Tapp stance. Stand with your feet hip width apart and toes forward.

Bend your knees. Tuck your butt under and press your lower back against your hand at the same time you push into your stomach with your other hand. You should feel your abdominal core

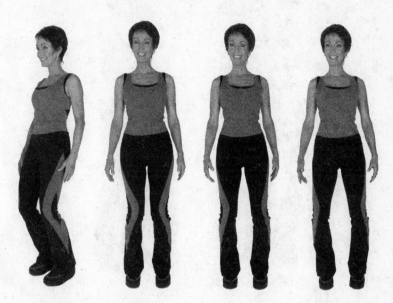

Photo 2

muscles tighten, as well as your hip and gluteal muscles. Now lift your ribs and align your shoulders with your hips, but do not arch your back. (See Photo 1.)

By now you should feel every muscle activate throughout your body. Push your knees out toward your little toes. (See Photo 2.) In addition to feeling increased muscle activation on the outside of your hip and thighs, you should feel deep lower abdominal activation (transverse abdominus).

Proceed to step 2.

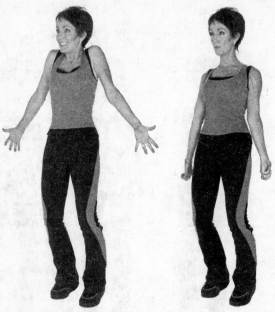

Photo 3

Step 2

WARM-UP SHOULDERS WITH TRAP/LAT STRETCHES

Inhale deeply and lift your shoulders up as high as you can with your arms straight down, palms forward, and fingers stretching wide (counts 1 to 4). (See Photo 3.) Then exhale deeply while your hands reach down close to the sides of your body with fingers folded and thumbs pointing back (counts 5 to 8). Repeat for a total of four sets, eight counts each.

Proceed to step 3.

Step 3

WARM-UP SPINE WITH PROGRESSIVE TUCK, CURL, AND SCOOP

Push your hands into your knees with your thumb on the inside and fingers on the outside of each knee. While pushing, tuck your butt under and curl your back until your arms are straight. Inhale deeply during the curl (counts 1 to 4) and exhale as you reverse, scooping out your spine and arching your butt up (counts 5 to 8).

Repeat, but this time reach your shoulders up toward your ears during the tuck/curl aand stretch your chin up on when you scoop.

Repeat two more tuck, curl, and scoops but with the following variation:

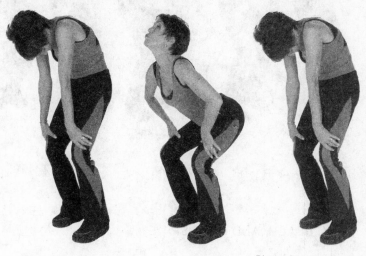

Photo 4

Tuck/curl with shoulders up (counts 1 and 2) and pull your shoulders back without bending your arms (counts 3 and 4). (See Photo 4.)

Then lift your shoulders up without bending your arms (counts 5 and 6) and scoop (counts 7 and 8).

Form check. Push thumbs and squeeze hands into your thighs to increase neurokinetic flow (mind-to-muscle transmission) during curls and aim your elbows forward during scoops. Keep your knees bent in KLT at all times with weight off the ball joint of your big toe.

Proceed to step 4.

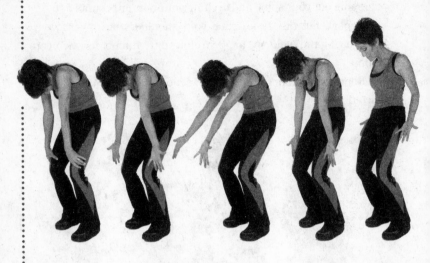

Photo 5

Step 4
TUCK, REACH, AND CURL SPINE

Inhale, tuck, and curl one more time without reaching shoulders up (counts 1 to 4), but flip your palms forward and tuck your butt under at the same time you reach down (counts 5 to 8) during exhale. Inhale again (counts 1 to 4), but this time during exhale, tuck and reach your arms forward (counts 5 to 8). Hold this position and inhale again (counts 1 to 3), then tuck and use your lats to pull your shoulders back (count 4) and continue to exhale as you roll your spine up one vertebra at a time (counts 5 to 8). (See Photo 5.)

Form check. Drag your little finger along the outside of your thighs, but bend your elbows and lift your ribs before you lift your chin. Keep your knees bent and pushing out at all times (KLT).

Proceed to step 5.

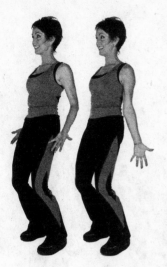

Step 5
TRAP/LAT SHOULDER ROLLS

Inhale as you reach your shoulders up (count 1), back (count 2), and down (count 3, hold 4) for a total of four sets, four counts each. (See Photo 6.)

Form check. Maintain lat activation and keep your hands below your waist or hips during the shoulder roll. Keep your thumbs turned back as far as you can and really reach up to release tension in your traps.

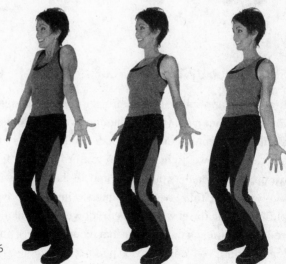

Photo 6

Most common mistake. Overreaching down can create imbalanced muscle activation in your shoulders, especially the traps.

Proceed to step 6.

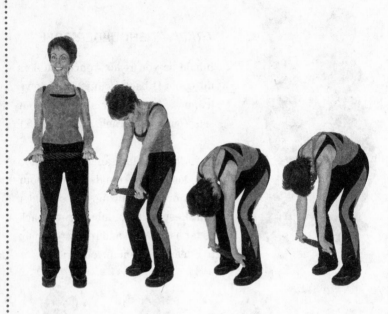

Step 6
SPINE ROLL-UP WITH TOWEL

Resume T-Tapp stance (bend it, tuck it, ribs up, knees out). Hold a towel with your palms up and thumbs away. Your wrists should be aligned with your shoulders. Inhale (counts 1 to 4), then during exhale, pull towel tight (counts 5 to 8).You should feel your ribs lift up, your shoulders pull back, and all the muscles in your back tighten. I call this leverage isometric muscle activation. Keep pulling on the towel while you curl down. Then inhale deep until you feel your back muscles stretch (counts 1 to 4), and exhale all the way until you feel your ribs pull together (counts 5 to 8). (See Photo 7.)

Form check. Keep your head relaxed and your knees bent and pushing out (KLT) at all times.

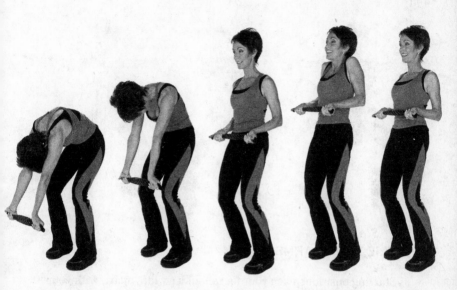

Photo 7

Inhale (counts 1 to 4) with your shoulders reaching up and maintain this position while you exhale (counts 5 to 8). Inhale again with your shoulders up (counts 1 to 4), butt tuck/curl, and bring your shoulders back down during exhale (counts 5 to 8). Inhale again (counts 1 to 4), but this time, tuck and reach out during exhale (counts 5 to 8). Inhale again while reaching (counts 1 to 4), but tuck and curl until the towel touches above your knees during exhale (counts 5 to 8). Keep tucking, curling, and pulling the towel while you curl up one vertebra at a time. Finish with four shoulder rolls reaching shoulders up (counts 1 and 2), back (count 3), and down (count 4).

Form check. Never release or relax towel. Keep it tight.

Drop towel, kick the legs several times to shake them out, and take a water break.

Proceed to step 7.

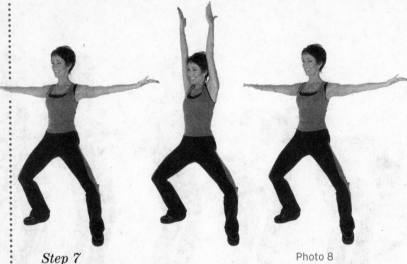

Photo 8

Step 7
PLIÉ SQUAT—ARMS UP

Starting position: place your feet shoulder width apart, with your toes turned out at a thirty-degree angle or less. Bend your knees, tuck your butt under to press your lower back flat, lift your ribs to activate your lats, and push your knees out until you feel your weight shift off the ball joint of your big toe. Your shoulders should be in alignment with or inside your heels and back in alignment with your hips. Now extend your arms out with your wrists, elbows, and shoulders in alignment. (See Photo 8.) Your palms should be up with your thumbs pointing back to your best ability. Your hands should be reaching out with the elbows locked.

Inhale deeply (counts 1 to 4) and exhale deeply (counts 5 to 8) with your arms extended two times.

Tuck a little bit more and bend your knees deeper as you extend your arms straight up (counts 1 and 2). Now reach your hands up and out until your arms are level with your shoulders with palms up and thumbs back (counts 3 and 4).

Repeat for a total of four sets, four counts each.

Proceed to step 8 without stopping.

Step 8
PLIÉ SQUAT–ARMS DOWN

Inhale again (counts 1 to 4) with your arms extended, then exhale while you lower them down (counts 5 to 8). Repeat.

Form check. Focus to keep your ribs up when your arms lower down and extend your hands out and up when you lift your arms to shoulder level (it should feel as if you are lifting something heavy).

Keep your arms at shoulder level. Inhale/exhale. Then repeat the same sequence with two counts at each position for a total of four sets, four counts each.

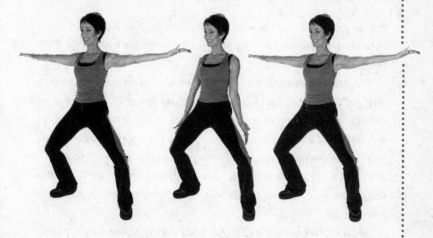

Photo 9

Lower arms (counts 1 and 2), and lift/extend your arms up (counts 3 and 4). (See Photo 9.)

Form check. Maintain the lower body position with knees out, shoulders back, and lower back flat (no arch) at all times.

Proceed to step 9 without stopping.

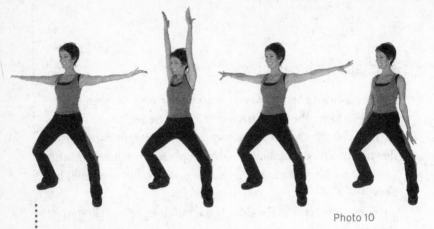

Photo 10

Step 9
PLIÉ SQUAT–FLIP SEQUENCE

Inhale (counts 1 to 4) and exhale (counts 5 to 8) with your arms extended, palms up, and thumbs back once before starting. (See Photo 10.)

Tuck and bend your knees deeper as you extend your arms straight up (counts 1 and 2), then lift your ribs and flip your palms down as you lower your arms to shoulder level in one count (count 3, hold count 4). Tuck and lift your ribs a little more as you lower your arms down in one count with palms facing inward (count 5, hold 6). Then lift your arms up to your shoulders (count 7) and flip your palms up (count 8). Repeat for a total of four sets, eight counts each.

Without stopping, repeat again, but with quick arm movement: arms up (counts 1 and 2), flip down (counts 3 and 4).

Form check. Tuck and press your lower back flat every time your arms go up, and lift your ribs each time your arms move up and down. Keep elbows straight.

Kick left and right legs four times to shake them out, alternate knee lifts four times, and take a break for water.

Proceed to step 10.

Step 10
PLIÉ SQUATS–REACH PULLS

Resume plié squat stance (shoulders back, ribs up, butt tucked, lower back pressed flat, and knees out). Place your arms into a big *W* position with your palms facing center and your fingers stretching wide. Now push your elbows forward and pull your hands back. You should feel ribs lift and every muscle in your upper back tighten. This push/pull action will also help you maintain correct linear alignment (wrists, elbows, and shoulders) as well as maximize mind-to-muscle activation. (See Photo 11.)

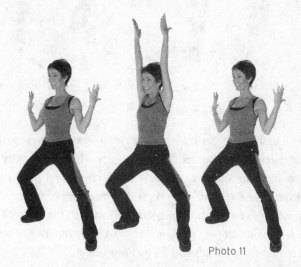

Photo 11

Inhale deeply and while you tuck, bend, and push your knees out more, extend your arms straight up (counts 1 to 4). Then, while exhaling, pull your arms back down into the *W* position with elbows forward and hands back in alignment with your shoulders (counts 5 to 8). Repeat.

Repeat again, but this time hold two counts in each position for a total of four sets, four counts each.

Proceed to step 11 without stopping.

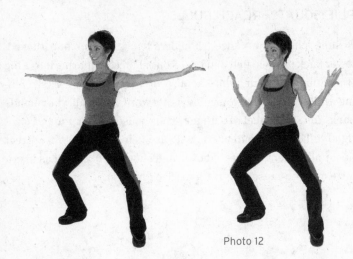

Photo 12

Step 11
PLIÉ SQUATS–LATERAL PULLS

While maintaining the plié squat position, extend your arms at shoulder level with palms up and fingers wide. Make sure that your wrist is in alignment with your shoulder and behind your ear. Inhale first (counts 1 to 4) while your arms are extended. Then, while exhaling, pull your elbows down to the sides of your body with your elbows pushing forward and your hands pulling back (counts 5 to 8). Repeat. (See Photo 12.)

Form check. Maintain alignment of your elbows and hands with your shoulders or ears while pulling into the *W* position, and exhale deep while you pull your ribs in.

Inhale again as you extend your arms back out in alignment with your shoulders (counts 1 and 2) and exhale while pulling them into the *W* position (counts 3 and 4) for a total of four sets, four counts each.

Proceed to step 12 without stopping.

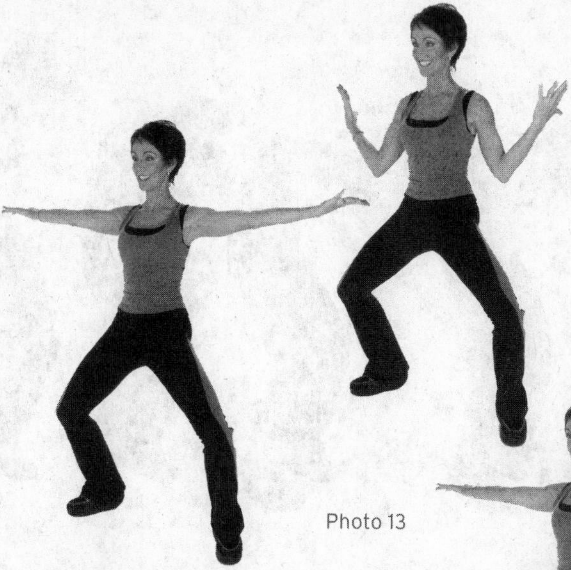

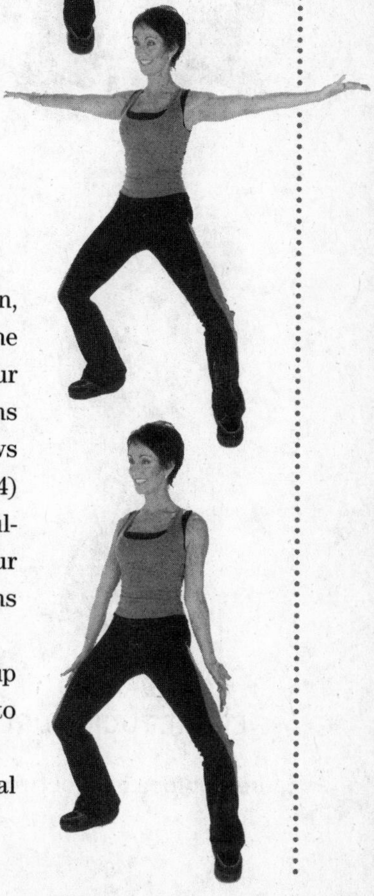

Photo 13

Step 12
PLIÉ SQUAT–LATERAL COMBO

While maintaining the plié squat position, focus on your form and continue to do the following combo sequence: extend your arms out at shoulder level with your palms up (count 1, hold 2). Then pull your elbows down into the *W* position (count 3, hold 4) and extend your arms back out at shoulder level (count 5, hold 6). Lower your arms with the elbows straight and palms up (count 7, hold 8). (See Photo 13.)

Form check. Always lift your ribs up when lowering your arms and pulling into the *W* position.

Repeat the combo sequence for a total of four sets, eight counts each.

Proceed to step 13.

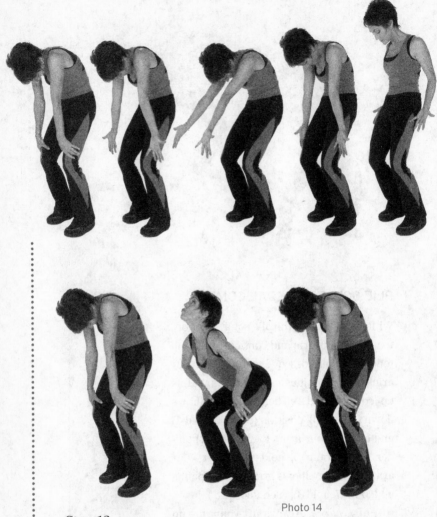

Photo 14

Step 13

REPEAT TUCK, CURL, AND SCOOP

Repeat for a total of two sets, eight counts each. (See Photo 14.)

Proceed to step 14.

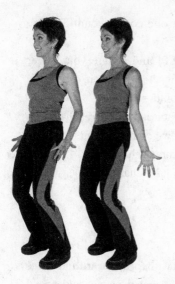

Step 14
REPEAT TUCK, REACH, AND ROLL

Repeat step 4 (Tuck, Reach, and Curl Spine) and finish with two shoulder rolls.

Form Check. Focus on activating your lats to pull your shoulders back as you roll up one vertebra at a time and keep knees out. (See Photo 15.)

Proceed to step 15.

Photo 15

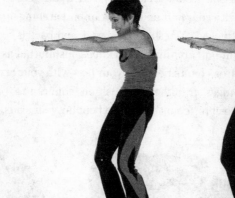

Step 15
STANDING LAT WARM-UP

Photo 16

While maintaining your lower body in the T-Tapp stance, extend your arms at shoulder level with hands together in the dive position. Inhale deeply (counts 1 to 4), then, while exhaling, tuck and reach straight out for three counts (counts 5 to 7). Lift your ribs and pull your shoulders back in one count (count 8). (See Photo 16.)

Form check. Keep knees out (KLT) and isolate your lower body position. Focus on upper body muscle activation, especially your lats, and keep your wrist and shoulder aligned.

Repeat, but change the count sequence as follows: reach for two counts (counts 1 and 2), pull back for two counts (counts 3 and 4). Repeat for a total of four sets, four counts each.

Proceed to step 16A without stopping.

Step 16A
OIL WELLS

Place your feet shoulder width apart with toes forward and knees bent pushing out. Assume a flat back position with your shoulders and back level with your hips and with your butt arching up toward the ceiling (not tucked). You should feel as if your back is scooping out.

Keep your butt arching up and knees pushing out as you reach/ pulse for three counts between your legs with your arms straight and hands together in the dive position (counts 1 to 3). Return to a flat back position (count 4) without bending your arms. (See Photo 17A.)

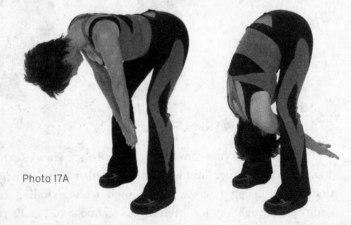

Photo 17A

Form check. Use your lats to pull your shoulders back to a flat back position. Additionally, your head should stay relaxed and your hands should stay together while reaching through your legs.

Repeat for a total of four sets, four counts each.

Proceed to step 16B without stopping.

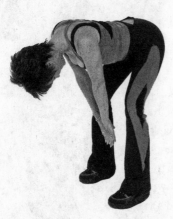 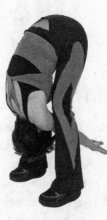

Step 16B
OIL WELLS

Continue the same movement, but change the sequence to single counts. Reach (count 1) and pull back (count 2). Do four sets, two counts each, for a total of eight counts. (See Photo 17B.)

Proceed to step 17.

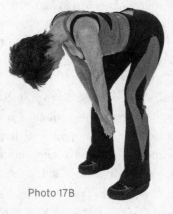

Photo 17B

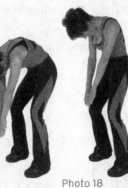

Photo 18

Step 17
OIL WELLS ROLL-UP

Inhale while maintaining the flat back position (counts 1 and 2). While keeping your knees out and your hands together in the dive position, reach down as you tuck your butt (counts 3 and 4), and slowly roll up one vertebra at a time (counts 5 to 8). Lift your head and your arms with bent elbows and do four arm pumps (counts 1 to 4). Finish with one big shoulder roll (counts 5 to 8). (See Photo 18.)

Form check. Keep your back muscles tight to help stabilize your shoulders when you pull your hands back above your head. It's important to keep your butt tucked and knees out too. (See Photo 19.)

Take a break for water and proceed to step 18.

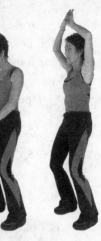

Photo 19

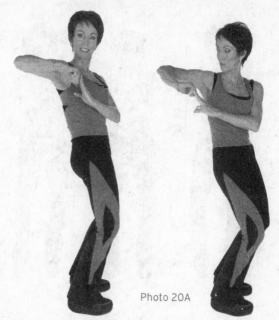

Photo 20A

Step 18
T-TAPP TWIST STRETCH

Resume the T-Tapp stance (toes forward, knees bent, butt tucked under, ribs up, shoulders back, and knees out in KLT). Place your right elbow up level with your shoulder or slightly higher with your wrist slightly lower. While keeping your left shoulder back in alignment with your hips, reach your left arm under your chest until your left fingertips are able to touch your right hand knuckles. It is important to lift your ribs and maintain isometric activation of your upper back and shoulder muscles at all times, especially the latissimus dorsi and traps. Not only will this accelerate results, it provides spinal support and helps offset muscle imbalance. (See Photo 20A.)

Inhale deeply and push your left knee out even more to help stabilize your hips while you exhale and push your right hand to twist and move your right elbow back as far as you can and hold four counts (counts 1 to 4). Relax and release your twist, but do

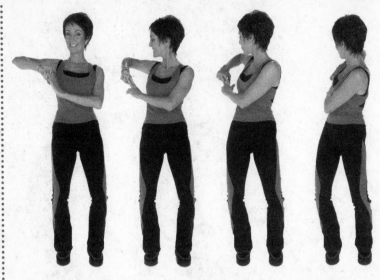

Photo 20B

not lower your right elbow or release your T-Tapp stance (counts 5 to 8). Then inhale deeper, but this time during the exhale, increase the intensity of your tuck, knees out and ribs up while you twist and look back as far as you can.

Form check. Really focus to maintain alignment of your right elbow to shoulder when twisting back. Try to pull your ribs together during the exhale and *never* allow your right elbow to drop lower than your shoulder.

Most common mistakes. Allowing your right elbow to drop below shoulder level and not keeping your butt tucked can create unsafe conditions for your spine. Allowing your left knee to release inward or your right elbow to reach too high will inactivate many muscles and lessen the effectiveness of this exercise. (See Photo 20B.)

Repeat the twist stretch to the other side with your left elbow up for a total of two sets, eight counts each.

Proceed to step 19.

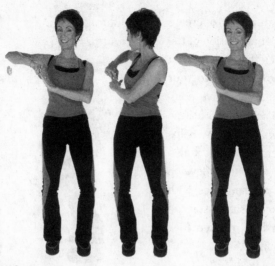

Step 19
T-TAPP TWIST SEQUENCE

Photo 20C

Twist your upper body to the right and pulse for three counts without moving your lower body. Then in one count, tuck, lift ribs, and twist quickly back to the front position (counts 1 to 4). Repeat (counts 5 to 8). (See Photo 20C.)

Reset your upper body position with the left elbow up and repeat the twist sequence to your left for a total of two sets, four counts each.

Continue doing two twisting sets per side for an overall total of four sets. Count one set as follows: Twist/pulse right (counts 1 to 3), tuck center (count 4), twist/pulse right again (counts 5 and 6), tuck center (count 7), switch arms (count 8). Repeat left. Repeat three more times for a total of four sets, eight counts each.

Form check. Keep pressing your hands together and try to maintain pressure between them during this exercise to maximize muscle activation. This will help keep your ribs up and create balanced isometric activation of your lats and oblique muscles.

Most common mistake. Having too wide a stance makes it

more difficult to create full fiber activation of the muscles that attach from your lower spine to your hip. Comprehensive, compound activation of these muscles not only helps protect your spine, it also helps your body develop more core muscles with greater density so you can lose inches quicker. (See Photo 21.)

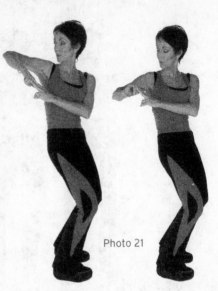

Photo 21

Proceed to step 20.

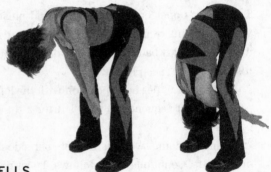

Step 20
REPEAT OIL WELLS, PART 1

Repeat two sets of step 16A (Oil Wells, Part 1), four counts each for a total of eight counts.

Inhale deeply until you feel your ribs expand and exhale deeply until your feel your ribs pull together without relaxing your shoulders forward. (See Photo 22.)

Proceed to step 21.

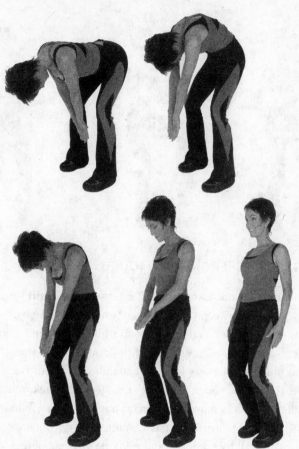

Step 21
LAT ROLL-UP

Photo 23

This sequence is like step 17, but with extra focus on using your shoulder and upper back muscles to initiate the roll-up. Also it's important to keep tucking and reaching down while rolling up to maximize stretch and muscle activation of all your back muscles, especially the lats. Then finish with one big shoulder roll and take a break for water before starting step 22—Hoedowns. (See Photo 23.)

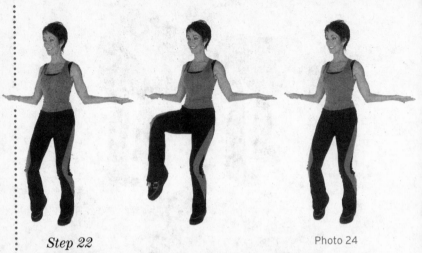

Step 22

Photo 24

HOEDOWNS–FRONT LIFT/TOUCH

Starting position: assume the T-Tapp stance, but shift your weight to your left leg. Keep your left knee bent in the KLT position, your butt tucked under, and your ribs up while you extend your hands out to the sides of your body with palms up and thumbs back. Now push your elbows forward and pull your hands back to your best ability. You should feel your shoulders pull back, your ribs lift higher, and every muscle tighten in your upper back. Inhale deeply until you feel your ribs expand, and exhale deeply until you feel your ribs pull together without relaxing your shoulders forward. Now that every muscle in your body is isometrically activated, you're ready to start.

Lift your right knee up in alignment with your right shoulder (count 1), then tap your toes to the floor (count 2). Repeat for a total of four lifts and four taps (8 counts). (See Photo 24.)

Form check. Try not to move your upper body when lifting your knee. Keep your butt tucked and your left knee bent in KLT at all times. Also, point your toe with each lift to increase activation of the abdominal muscles.

Proceed to step 23 without stopping.

Step 23
HOEDOWNS—SIDE LIFT/TOUCH

Without stopping, lift your right knee up and out to the right side as you bring your right hand across your body to the left (count 1) and tap your toes to the floor (count 2). Repeat for a total of four lifts and taps (eight counts). (See Photo 25.)

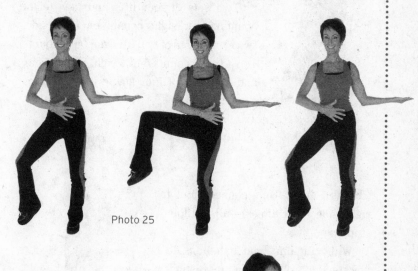

Photo 25

Form check. Linear alignment is important during lifts and taps. In addition to aiming your knee toward your shoulder while lifting, keep your ankle in alignment with your knee. (See Photo 26A.)

Photo 26A

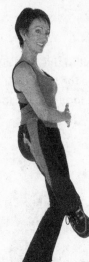

Most common mistake. Allowing your foot to shift out of alignment while lifting your knee (front and side) creates inactivation of the abdominal muscles and lessens effectiveness. (See Photo 26B.)

Repeat front and side lift/touch sequence as follows:

Two sets of four lifts and taps (eight counts front, eight counts on right side, twice), two sets of two lifts and taps (counts 1 to 4 front, counts 5 to 8 right side, twice), and two sets of four single lifts and taps

Photo 26B

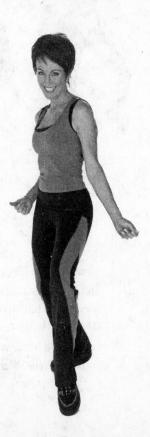

(counts 1 and 2 front, counts 3 and 4 right side, four times)—all without stopping.

While inhaling and exhaling, do one shoulder roll back and reset starting position to repeat the same sequence on the other side (two sets of four, two sets of two, and one set of four single lifts and taps with left knee).

Inhale deeply, exhale deeper, and repeat the entire sequence (right side, then left side) for a total of two sets of Hoedowns.

"YOU DID IT!"

Now take a break for water and *have a great day.*

A Final Note about Exercise

One word of caution: don't go overboard with exercise. I realize that this is not a problem for many of us (myself included!), but for those of you who throw yourselves into fitness, sports, or exercise, keep in mind that overexercising can create added stress, which can cause inflammation, deplete your adrenal glands, and further aggravate your hormonal imbalances.

Acupuncturist and Chinese medicine practitioner Dr. Jocelyne Eberstein has some thoughts:

> Excessive exercise stresses the adrenals, and causes inflammation. You can't go to the gym, work out ninety minutes, and not stress your adrenals. So it's best to divide up your exercise, allowing time to rest in between.

How will you know if you are overexercising?

- You feel fatigued to the point of needing a nap after an exercise session.
- You have excessive pain during or after exercise.
- You feel flulike symptoms after exercise.
- You are sluggish in the hours or day after exercise.
- You feel mentally exhausted in the hours or day after exercise.
- You are quick to develop aches, pains, and injuries during and after exercise and are slower to recover.

Remember that whatever exercise you choose, in your forties and beyond, it's easier to injure your body than when you were younger. You may find that joints and muscles are not as strong or as flexible as they once were. So when you're getting back into exercise, remember some safety tips:

- Always warm up and stretch before exercising.
- Try for moderate activity every day if possible, rather than being a "weekend warrior."
- Take lessons, or work with a trainer, to learn the proper form and how to prevent injury.
- Balance your exercise program with a combination of cardio/aerobics, strength, and flexibility cross-training to work out the entire body and avoid injuries due to overuse.

If you just can't bear the thought of any exercise program, then put on a pair of sneakers and, as Dr. Teitelbaum said, "Go outside, get sunshine, and get walking!"

chapter 9

The Role of Mind, Body,
AND SPIRIT

> You must learn to be still in the midst of activity
> and to be vibrantly alive in repose.
>
> —*Indira Gandhi*

Going through perimenopause into menopause with the ability to weather symptoms depends on a lot more than just medicine, herbs, and lifestyle issues like diet and exercise. It depends on your attitude.

If you are someone who views health in a holistic way, then you understand that mind and body are linked. But even if you don't have a holistic perspective, you can still understand the importance of attitude on your hormonal health.

Even in ancient times, there was the belief that we needed three different doctors for healing: the "knife" doctor (for surgery), the "herb" doctor (for medications), and the "word" doctor.

From today's scientific standpoint, the "word" doctors are not just psychiatrists and psychologists, but neuroendocrinologists, who study the interactions between the nervous system and the endocrine system. Neuroendocrinology is the science of mind–body medicine, in a way, and it has grown as scientists have increasingly recognized that the release of hormones is closely controlled by the brain and that emotions and attitudes affect hormones.

Take adrenaline, the fight-or-flight hormone, for example. Simply thinking about something you're afraid of or a stressful situation can cause your body to start pumping out adrenaline, which then raises your heart rate and blood pressure. So mind affects body. Similarly, a new mother who even looks at a photo of her baby usually experiences a release of oxytocin, a hormone that causes a feeling of well-being and an increase in milk supply. Again, mind affects body.

In talking with some of the nation's leading experts on hormones, menopause, and thyroid disease, I discovered some wonderful recommendations for bringing a mind–body component into your overall approach to hormonal imbalances.

Have a Positive Attitude

Around the world, menopause is associated with uncomfortable symptoms. But for many women, menopause is also a positive, life-affirming time.

If you're just entering perimenopause, it's hard to look toward menopause with anything but trepidation, and asking you to have a positive attitude may sound a bit nuts. But you may be surprised to learn that a North American Menopause Society survey of women ages fifty to sixty-five found that the majority of women feel that this is the *best* time of life. It's a time when women report feeling confident, fulfilled, free to pursue their interests and passions. As many as one in three women will go through menopause without any particularly troublesome symptoms.

Holistic physician Tieraona Low Dog explains:

It's rare to find women who think they will go through menopause without problems. And yet, in my practice, about 30 percent of women *never* have a hot flash. But we don't study the women who go through menopause without symptoms. We don't study the group of women who transition with very little turmoil.

My own grandmother, who is in her nineties, went through menopause at a time forty years ago when hormones were just coming on the scene, and she didn't take them. I asked her about her menopause, and honestly, she's not quite sure what I'm asking her. "I remember when my periods stopped, I did have a few hot flashes," she said. But she doesn't view it as a problem, and she didn't "do" anything for them. "I had to change my shirt," she says. Or, "In bed, I'd get hot and had to kick off the covers sometimes. Some nights it bothered me a bit, but it didn't last forever." She's very matter of fact about it.

If you watch television or read magazines, you may think that every menopausal woman is walking around having constant hot flashes. The reality, however, is that many women are going through menopause with a fairly matter-of-fact attitude about it all. You'll probably hear complaints from the women in your life who are having some menopausal difficulties. Yet how many women you know are going through menopause right now, but you don't even know about it, because they're taking the symptoms in stride?

It's helpful to think of how you felt during the other major period of hormonal fluctuation for women: puberty. Most of us didn't one day just develop breasts and body hair and start menstruating on a perfect twenty-eight-day schedule, with no premenstrual syndrome (PMS) and no cramps. Truthfully, it was probably far more erratic. Some of us watched as one breast grew more quickly than the other. We had hormonal mood swings, and eventually, we started getting a period. But it usually took many months, or even several years, for our period to become regular. Some of us discovered that PMS and cramps were also part of the picture.

We don't rush in to medicate every symptom of puberty. In turn, some practitioners suggest that we don't need to view every symptom of menopause as a problem that requires medication.

Dr. Low Dog explains:

When women ask me, "What should I do for menopause" I often ask, "What did you do for your puberty? How did you get through it?" Most women are floored by these questions. The good news is, you successfully navigated through puberty. I'm confident you'll be able to navigate through menopause without much difficulty. Most women reflect upon that . . . they know it didn't happen overnight, it was a several-year transition.

Holistic health expert Dr. Annemarie Colbin agrees:

We need to stop thinking about having "hormone problems." It's not a problem or a medical condition, and you're not sick.

Stefanie Rotsaert, a thyroid patient and founder of a successful patient support group in New Jersey, found that a positive attitude was very helpful during menopause. Says Rotsaert:

I always try to believe in the best. I believe if you feel that way, it is. My main symptom was hot flashes, and occasionally I had some night sweats. I didn't think negatively, I assumed that was what it was and went with it. Many people have a negative attitude . . . they feel that they are the only person with a medical problem, the only person suffering. But I think with a negative attitude, the problem gets worse. Doctors all notice my positive attitude. I have a lot of energy and a lot of enthusiasm, and, you know, I think it's contagious!

Use Affirmations and Self-Hypnosis

One of the most effective ways to communicate mind to body is through positive affirmations, or self-hypnosis. When you think of hypnosis, you may have images of hypnotists on stage, making audience members cluck like chickens. But that's not what hypnosis is about.

Osteopathic physician Scott Kwiatkowski has an interesting way of explaining the mind–body connection:

> There is you, and there is your body. You need to realize that you have a relationship with your body. Think of your body as your best friend, who loves you but doesn't speak any English. You speak to your body with your thoughts; your body speaks back to you with images, feelings, symptoms, and pain.

Noted guided imagery therapist Belleruth Naparstek explains that the brain doesn't know the difference between something you actually see and something you imagine. So your body can respond as strongly to an image or a thought as to the real thing. Naparstek has told *Prevention* magazine that guided imagery helps you "get in under your mind's radar" so that you can persuade your body to do something.

> It may be to increase brain chemicals that make you feel calm and centered, decrease hormones that make you hungry, change the levels of biochemical components in your bloodstream that affect blood sugar, even build more immune system cells to fight everything from cancer to the common cold.

Think of self-hypnosis techniques as a way of taking positive images of your body, and the hormonal changes you are facing, and translating them into a language your body understands.

Steven Gurgevich, PhD, is a clinical psychologist and a foremost expert in medical hypnosis and mind–body medicine. He is director of the Mind–Body Clinic at the University of Arizona's College of Medicine, where he teaches mind–body medicine to physicians at Dr. Andrew Weil's Program in Integrative Medicine. Dr. Gurgevich feels that how we think about menopause, and ourselves during menopause, plays a critical role in how we feel. According to Dr. Gurgevich:

> We know that the hormonal changes are happening in the brain—for example, as estrogen drops, the body "thinks" we're cooling down, so it has to heat us up again with hot flashes. If it's happening in the brain, why not approach it in the brain?

It's one thing to tell ourselves we need to be positive, or to have affirmation, but it's another thing to convince our body that we truly believe them. This is where self-hypnosis comes in. Says Dr. Gurgevich:

> In my work with mind–body approaches and hypnosis—whether it's visualization, guided imagery, or autogenics—when you combine that approach with a hypnotic state, and you have the robustness and power of excluding distractions, the body really gets the message, faster and better. The key is to help the conscious mind—the critical evaluator—to step aside enough to let the mind–body connection really work. It takes some repetition, to replace old ideas with new positive ideas, but it can work if we are willing to stay with it.

According to Dr. Gurgevich, studies have shown that there are a number of benefits of self-hypnosis for women in perimenopause/menopause, including

- Reduced intensity and frequency of hot flashes
- Reduced reaction to hot flashes
- Reduced night sweats
- Improved mood
- Less anxiety

Dr. Gurgevich has found that the more a woman can have positive thoughts about her body and menopause, the more successful and comfortable her menopause. But Dr. Gurgevich emphasizes that affirmations used in self-hypnosis must emphasize the truth. They must be honest.

To explore self-hypnosis for yourself, you may want to try the following brief session developed by Dr. Gurgevich:

Think of your "thinking mind" (conscious mind) as a magnifying glass that will concentrate the energy and intention of your affirmative statements. If you like, think of your mind as a clear, still pool that is concentrating the sunlight to nourish the plants growing at the bottom of the pool. In other words, be creative and imaginative. The intention and energy of these affirmations are being absorbed by your subconscious mind (that's the mind of your body), which can perform all of the physical functions automatically or autonomically. You don't have to repeat them more than once or twice, but it is important to let yourself believe in what you are saying to yourself (either silently within or aloud). You can create images to match the statements and positive outcomes if you like.

My body is performing naturally and in harmony with the time and nature of health.

Each day I experience greater ease and comfort as my body is adjusting to the next healthy phase of my life.

Experiencing menopause is letting me learn better ways to reduce stress and increase my pleasures in life.

My female organs are vitally healthy and making comfortable adjustments for me now.

With each day I am achieving healthy menopause with comfort, peace, poise, and confidence that all is well.

I have a powerful connection between my healthy loving thoughts and my body's physical responses.

My positive and loving thoughts of self resonate throughout my body, and menopause is now easier and easier to experience as the natural process it is.

When estrogen levels drop, my body is learning that this is normal, and my temperature remains comfortably normal too.

My body sleeps me restfully, comfortably, and gently as it so quietly continues a healthy journey through menopause.

I am now more relaxed and at ease with my body, and I am grateful that my body receives and believes my thoughts of comfort.

Dr. Gurgevich has created a self-hypnosis audio program featuring these and many more affirmations for perimenopause and menopause. Information on that program, as well as his many incredible self-hypnosis resources, is available in the book's Web site www.menopausethyroid.com.

If you are interested in working with a medical hypnotist personally, Dr. Gurgevich says the general rule is that you don't want a practitioner to treat something with hypnosis unless he or she is qualified to treat it *without* hypnosis. So always work with a qualified medical or mental health care professional who is certified by the American Society of Clinical Hypnosis.

Redirect and Rebalance Your Life Energy

One of the ways to have a positive attitude through perimenopause and beyond is to realize that at menopause, your energy can be redirected to other areas. Dr. Tieraona Low Dog calls it "your reproductive/potential-of-life energy," and whether or not you've had children, it's a time when many women find themselves shifting their creative energy toward new interests and endeavors.

This is why, says Dr. Low Dog, many menopausal women may take up a new hobby, a new career, or do something they've put off. Holistic physician Dr. Molly Roberts has some thoughts:

One of the most important things is to relax around menopause. This is a natural, normal life transition. Even hot flashes are more significant if you tighten up around the symptoms. Physically and emotionally, anything not in balance will start showing up and making itself known. To help stay balanced, you can ask yourself, "What am I here to do on this planet?" Then take a life review of what is and is not working. Step into the joy, the passion, the juiciness of your own life. Then symptoms won't be as predominant in your life.

Dr. Jan Nicholson, a holistic therapist, has some thoughts on how to focus on the positive, and redirect creative energy:

The important thing is to find what gives us joy and to do more of that, to notice our feelings as important indicators about what we need, and about changes we might want to make in our lives, rather than seeing feelings as things to avoid. As a transition time, it can be a great time to see a psychotherapist or a life coach for support as we go through the changes and to find excitement within to start thinking outside the box about our lives. Whether we see someone for help with this or not, there are great questions we can ask ourselves and then live our way into the answers. For example: How do we want to enter this creative phase of life? What are things we've always wanted to do but haven't yet done? If we open to inspiration, what new things might come to us that we have never even considered before? Since it is a transition time, and changes are occurring outside of our control, it is empowering to consider it as a time to make our lives a more true reflection of ourselves.

Dr. Molly Roberts says that balance is essential:

Biochemistry won't allow you to be dishonest with yourself. Things out of balance will be in your face. During perimeno- pause and menopause, you have the potential to look at what is out of balance and create the life that feels most integrated with you as a human being. If you medicate that away, you may not have the chance to find outlets for your nurturing and creativity, you may not find your own power.

Choose Your Health Direction

One helpful mind–body approach toward menopause is to consider it a time to evaluate your health and pay attention to how you feel and what you can and should do to enjoy good health for many years to come. Menopause may also be a good time to finally learn balance in your life and how to set time aside to care for your own health.

Menopause is a good time to take stock of your health habits and decide about how best to eat, exercise, and take care of yourself in order to enjoy good health moving forward.

Ob-gyn and North American Menopause Society spokesperson Dr. Jan Shifren feels that taking care of ourselves is especially im- portant in perimenopause/menopause.

Perimenopause often takes place during a difficult time in a woman's life—her children are teenagers or young adults, and her parents are aging. It's physiologically a challenge, like ado- lescence, but at the same time, women are dealing with other baggage. A woman may be focusing on her husband's midlife crisis, or daughter's first baby, or have an elderly mother needing care. Women have to be prepared for the fact that there will be a lot of demands—physically and in terms of daily life—and be prepared to take care of themselves as well during this time. I often hear women say, "I don't exercise because I'm so busy taking care of . . . ," and this is the time when women *most* need to set aside that time to take care of themselves. If you have menopausal symptoms and they're bothersome, treat them. But your major goal is to view menopause as a time to reassess your health as you're getting older.

Therapist Dr. Jan Nicholson also feels that part of this health approach is to make time for stress management. According to Nicholson:

The most useful stress management approaches would be those tried-and-true ones that you have used earlier in life. If you haven't been pursuing stress management before, then consider taking a yoga or tai chi class, going to a meditation center, and making that a regular part of your life. Meditation, tai chi, and yoga are highly beneficial for having greater relaxation overall and enhanced peace of mind; they are also highly effective at reducing anxiety. And anxiety is one of the biggest symptoms I see in women who are perimenopausal/menopausal. Exercise is great for improving mood. Other possibilities would be having a massage, journaling, using relaxation techniques, taking bubble baths if you enjoy them, listening to soothing music, listening to guided imagery CDs, taking time in nature. It is a personal thing, whatever helps you to feel better, more relaxed.

Cultivate Friendships and Wisdom

Every woman practitioner I spoke with in researching this book emphasized the importance of connecting with other women during this important time of our life. Whether we forge new friendships and reconnect with existing ones, connect with more wise women in our lives, or make wisdom a personal goal, the period of perimenopause and menopause is the time when we really need our friends more than ever before.

Holistic physician Molly Roberts says that women may even want to establish rituals:

I have recommended that women get together with others—their peers—to start those rituals, when one friend is going into perimenopause, or when they're in menopause, to actually celebrate. Get your friends together, talk, kvetch, laugh, and mark the occasion with some sort of ritual or ceremony that commemorates stepping over that threshold. You'll find that some friends are further along, some are watching from the sidelines, but we can all start being helpful to each other.

Dr. Jan Nicholson feels that, in her experience both as a woman and as a clinician, women do not share about menopause with each other nearly enough.

Most women I know rely on their doctors and not much else to weather menopause. Part of that reluctance might be due to the stigma, for instance, not wanting others to know you have aged to that point, and not wanting to possibly face judgments or fearfulness from others. But it would be great for us to rely on our friends and acquaintances more, to have those open conversations. To check in with each other about symptoms we might be having in common could help relieve that sense that we are not alone in the process. For those who welcome a more formal way of joining together, there are workshops for menopausal women, and in some places, there are support groups.

Dr. Tieraona Low Dog believes that wisdom is an important goal at this time.

Some people refer to the postmenopausal years as the "crone" years. While I know how positively the word *crone* is intended, the word itself does have baggage for some people. I prefer "wisdom years."

Dr. Annemarie Colbin suggests that we should be open to the idea of finding other, wise women to help guide us in perimenopause and menopause. Says Colbin:

> We need to enjoy our wisdom years. And to help find one to guide you, I suggest that you put it in your mind that you would like to meet a wise older woman, and someone will show up. Wise older women don't go around saying, "I'm a wise old woman." They don't market themselves. But they show up when you need them.

Dr. Colbin is right. It became clear to me, as I encountered (in many cases, purely by chance) so many amazingly wise women, including, I might add, Dr. Colbin herself, who I was lucky enough to be able to call upon for advice and information as I wrote this book.

Recharge with the Heart

Osteopathic physician Scott Kwiatkowski says one of the most important things we can do during perimenopause/menopause is to get out of our heads and recharge—with the heart, not the head. According to Dr. Kwiatkowski, we need to calm the sympathetic nervous system, that part of our autonomic nervous system that is always activated and responds with a fight-or-flight reaction during times of stress.

> When the brain is always leading, you can't stop thinking, and this contributes to feeling stressed and depressed. Drugs and alcohol don't work. The key is getting "out of the mind." You can try gentle movement and physical exercise like yoga, tai chi,

walking, and swimming. Reconnecting with a spouse or lover is also an important part of recharging. Savor the food you're eating, the smells around you, the feeling of swimming, the receiving or giving of a massage to someone you love. You want to appreciate the feelings and get out of your head.

One of the basic ways we can do this, according to Dr. Kwiatkowski, is family massage, a suggestion we have instituted in my own family. In our hectic lives, it's a way that we can take time out to physically connect with each other, adults and children. Several times a week, we try to make time for even a few minutes to massage each other gently. It doesn't have to be skilled—even gentle rubbing, or rocking, or putting a soft hand on the back.

Says Dr. Kwiatkowski:

> And when you're done, everyone says thank you. It's a wonderful exchange, and even five minutes is a gift to each other. It's something to look forward to and count on.

Communicate with Your Partner

Communication applies not only to friends but also to partners and spouses.

Marisol was diagnosed with both perimenopause and thyroid problems at the same time, and they came after a period of upheaval with her partner.

> It's proved to be an emotional roller coaster at home with fluctuating moods and zip sex drive. My partner and I have had many problems and almost broke up several times because no one could explain what was wrong with me, so he interpreted it all as my emotional withdrawal from him because I didn't care about him anymore. Utter rubbish, is what I told him, and I became determined to get to the bottom of what was wrong with

me, so diagnosis worked like marriage therapy in a way, because once he knew it wasn't really "me," we began to work together to get to the bottom of this condition.

According to Dr. Jan Nicholson, talking to your partner or spouse is important.

If he's open to it, it might be good to give him something to read, a book, or provide him with more information online. Many men have heard stories about menopause and seem to worry that it is like PMS on steroids, so information about the reality is reassuring. It's good for the woman to share what symptoms she is having, and to share how he might be supportive. When I went through menopause, I had anxiety for the only time in my life, and it was associated with driving. I had difficulty being a passenger and needed to be in the driver's seat. I have heard this one from a number of women. So, using that as an example, we worked it out that I would always be the driver until that symptom diminished. (It took about six months.) There are other issues that come up that can be handled with humor, such as women throwing off all the covers at night, and husbands winding up having piles of sheets, blankets, and comforters on them. Or women suddenly no longer wanting to cuddle during the night because they get too hot from the body heat of their husbands. It is these kinds of everyday issues that are good to talk about, and it can be done in a way that both people can actually enjoy the conversation.

Breathe

It goes by a variety of names. In yoga, it's pranayama, the art and science of breathing. In marketing language, it's Breathercise or Oxycise. Some diet centers even incorporate it into their programs. Whatever you call it, a program of deep breathing exercises, designed to take in more oxygen and release more carbon dioxide with each breath, seems to help people in a number of ways.

For example, breathing experts point to numerous health benefits of systematic breathing practice, including increased oxygen delivery to the cells, which helps provide sufficient energy to fuel metabolism, improve digestion, lessen fatigue, improve energy, reduce stress, and relax. There are even studies demonstrating that certain types of breathing can reduce hot flashes. Learning how to breathe doesn't cost a thing. All you need is some air and a pair of lungs to start.

Acupuncturist Dr. Jocelyne Eberstein feels that breathing exercises are important, because "it's one way to add energy to the body besides food."

If you're interested in trying out better breathing for yourself, you can start by learning deep abdominal breathing. Here's a simple breathing exercise to try:

Lie on your back, body relaxed. Put your hand on your abdomen. Take a deep, slow breath through your nose, filling your belly, so your hand rises. Then exhale slowly, letting all the air out of your belly. Inhale again, filling the abdomen until your hand rises. Again, exhale. Feel the breath energy rising from the abdomen to the throat and back down again to the abdomen.

You can start practicing this deep, abdominal breathing anywhere: sitting in the car, waiting in line, standing in the shower. It's a first step toward incorporating deep breathing into your daily life. Several times a day, stop and just focus on your breathing. Take a few deep abdominal breaths. Every time you feel tired, try taking five deep abdominal breaths. See if these ventures in breathing practice help you feel a bit more energetic and alert.

Dr. Scott Kwiatkowski has some thoughts on why breathing is so important for women in perimenopause and menopause:

Proper breathing massages all the organs. And the point where the ribs meet the lower back is an area that particularly affects the ovaries. If you practice full abdominal breathing, this area is freed up, and blood supply to the ovaries is improved.

There are studies that have shown that abdominal breathing can substantially reduce hot flashes and help reduce their severity.

Abdominal breathing can be modified into a relaxation-style breathing exercise that is explained by noted holistic physician Dr. Andrew Weil. Holistic nutritionist Irma Jennings finds that her clients especially like Dr. Weil's breathing technique. Says Jennings:

During this time of what feels like disharmony, bringing awareness into your life through a meditative practice is most rewarding. It could be as simple as taking five deep cleansing breaths several times a day. My clients particularly benefit from Dr. Andrew Weil's breathing technique. This technique can be incorporated before your meals or anytime during the day whenever you feel emotionally, physically, or mentally fatigued or stressed.

To do Dr. Weil's 4-7-8 technique, put the tip of your tongue on the gum tissue right behind your front teeth. Exhale through your mouth with a whoosh, to a count of eight. Close your mouth and inhale quietly through your nose, counting to four. Hold your breath for a count of seven. Exhale completely through your mouth, making a whooshing sound to the count of eight. Continue for four cycles, keeping your tongue in the same position.

Irma Jennings suggests practicing this technique every day:

Use it whenever anything upsetting happens . . . *before* you react. Use it whenever you are aware of internal tension. Use it to help you fall asleep. This exercise cannot be recommended too highly. Everyone can benefit from it.

Note: Dr. Andrew Weil has a wonderful audio CD, *Breathing: The Masterkey to Self Healing/Meditation for Optimum Health*, that teaches eight different specialized breathing techniques. It's an excellent resource for anyone who wants to learn effective breathwork techniques.

Make a Spiritual Connection/Meditate

Finally, I think it's important to discuss the need for a spiritual connection. I'm not saying that you need to be religious, although for some people, religious practice, prayer, and regular attendance at a church, synagogue, temple, or mosque are clearly effective ways to achieve inner peace, a sense of well-being, a healthier feeling of calm, and a connection to God, the universe, or the divine.

But you do not need to be religious in order to be spiritual.

Spirituality can be expressed through a commitment to personal growth and development, through finding and practicing activities that make you feel fulfilled. You can volunteer for charitable groups that focus on helping people in need or making positive changes in the world. Attend spirituality workshops or retreats. Keep a spiritual journal, to note your goals and observations about your spiritual journey.

One of the most effective ways to foster a mind–body–spirit connection is meditation. According to the Center for Integrative Medicine at Thomas Jefferson University Hospital in Philadelphia, meditation training can help you cope with stress, have an improved sense of well-being, reduce body tension, and increase clearness of thinking, all effects that benefit the immune system. Meditation can help patients with chronic illnesses—including thyroid problems—to reduce symptoms and improve quality of life. Meditation has also been able to lower blood pressure, help clear up skin problems, and increase melatonin levels. Researchers have established by using magnetic resonance imaging (MRI) that meditation actually activates certain structures in the brain that control the autonomic nervous system.

I have found a variety of meditation approaches incredibly helpful in my own efforts to foster spirituality. In particular, I like the following audio programs:

Meditation for Beginners, by Jack Kornfield

How to Meditate, with Pema Chodron

Meditation in a New York Minute, by Mark Thornton

Another wonderful tool to aid in learning and practicing meditation and relaxation breathing is a fantastic product called *Healing Rhythms*, from Wild Divine. *Healing Rhythms* is an inexpensive biofeedback program and system that easily attaches to your home computer or laptop and offers interactive training on how to use your body's own signals (heart rate and so on) to monitor physical and emotional reactions to stress. *Healing Rhythms* features three prominent mind–body experts—Deepak Chopra, Dean Ornish, and Andrew Weil—who teach you using more than thirty different breathing and meditation exercises.

You can boost energy, reduce stress, reduce anxiety and depression, and, surprisingly, improve specific symptoms such as interrupted sleep and insomnia, urinary incontinence, headaches, and high blood pressure.

The way it works is that by providing you with physiological information, such as heart rate or body temperature, that you might not normally be aware of, you learn which types of activities—certain breathing, relaxation, and meditation patterns—can bring about specific and measurable changes in your physical response.

More information on *Healing Rhythms* is featured in Appendix A.

Laugh!

Dee Adams, founder of the terrific Minnie Pauz menopause site, www.MinniePauz.com, believes that humor can also be a wonderful coping strategy during menopause.

Dee says she was always a fan of the cartoon "Cathy," and she felt a similar approach was needed for women in menopause. Dee had never drawn a cartoon before she picked up her pen, and spent several years learning how to cartoon, just so she could create cartoons about the character she now calls her alter ego, "Minnie Pauz," the woman going through menopause. Dee is the creator of the wonderful cartoons featured in the beginning of the book.

Says Dee:

> I'm very serious about using humor to get through this process. As we all know, it's not just the menopause symptoms, but some underlying fears of aging that attack our self-worth. Laughter has been proven to physically improve our health. Sometimes it just has to be shoved in our faces before we remember to use it!

Dee's Minnie Pauz Web site is a popular destination for menopausal women, with a steady stream of Dee's new cartoons exploring the funny side of menopause, jokes about menopause, and a friendly support forum where women can share information and support. But the underlying theme of everything Dee does is that we are all in this together, and if we can laugh, it makes it that much easier. And I agree.

chapter 10

Solving Persistent
SYMPTOMS

The woman who is willing to make that change must
become pregnant with herself, at last.

—*Ursula Le Guin*

Sleep Problems and Fatigue

Even with optimal thyroid treatment, hormone therapy, and diet,
exercise, and lifestyle changes, you may still find that your most
troublesome continuing symptom is fatigue. You may feel as if you're
waking unrefreshed or as if you can't get through the day without a
nap. What else can you do?

First, you need to be sure that you are getting enough sleep. That
means eight hours for most of us—not seven, not six, but at least
eight hours. Many women tell me they are exhausted and have no
idea what to do about it, but when I ask them about their sleep habits, they are almost always trying to get by while chronically sleep
deprived, getting far less than eight hours a night. (According to the
National Sleep Foundation, one in three people in the United States
get six hours or less per night.) I am one of those people who do not

do well on less than seven and a half to eight hours. With young children, I got to a point where I was trying to get by on six hours a night and became exhausted. My first reaction was to blame my thyroid condition, but, no shock, when I made an effort to get back to eight hours a night, my energy dramatically improved. So, while proper treatment for hormonal imbalances is critical, don't even think about other ways to fight fatigue until you've taken this most basic first step of getting eight hours of sleep every night.

Physician and patient advocate Marie Savard agrees.

I have found that making a habit of getting seven to eight hours of sleep is a critical step—this will do far more to help than most things. Once you are sleeping more, you can add more difficult changes in small steps, such as improving your diet, drinking less caffeine, etc.

Dr. Tieraona Low Dog agrees that sleep is essential for women in menopause.

If you're not sleeping well, everything is worse. Hot flashes are worse, your body hurts more. Helping women sleep better makes so many symptoms a lot more tolerable.

If you are getting adequate sleep in terms of time, you may want to set up a video camera to tape yourself, or ask a partner or family member to do an informal "sleep study," to see if you are snoring or having episodes of sleep apnea where you briefly stop breathing. If any of these behaviors are observed, you should definitely have a formal, medically supervised sleep study. (Note: Apnea is more common in thyroid patients.)

If you're getting the hours in, but you're not getting quality sleep (you have a hard time falling asleep, you wake frequently, and so on), then you should start by practicing good sleep hygiene. This involves not using your bed as a place for work, television watching, or reading; establishing regular bedtime routines and schedules; getting enough exercise; limiting napping; avoiding stimulants before bedtime; avoiding food later in the evening; minimizing noise and light in the bedroom; keeping your bedroom cool; avoiding alcohol, caffeine, and nicotine; and other commonsense techniques.

The North American Menopause Society has some other recommendations to help with sleep:

- Add a light protein and carbohydrate bedtime snack to help with sleep (but keep in mind this is not optimal if you are trying to lose weight).
- Remember that the effects of caffeine can last as long as twenty hours, so watch the coffee drinks, colas, and various over-the-counter medications (such as weight-control aids, allergy and cold medications, and pain relievers) that are high in caffeine.
- If night sweats are particularly problematic, try special nightgowns and sheets with high-tech fabrics designed to keep you cooler and drier.

Ultimately, however, if you are unable to reestablish healthful sleeping patterns, you may wish to try a nonprescription sleep aid. These can include

- Over-the-counter drugs, such as diphenylhydramine (brand names Benadryl, Tylenol PM, and Excedrin PM) that are not habit forming. Note that some experts feel these products do not help with deep stage 4 sleep.
- Melatonin, particularly helpful if your body clock is off-kilter and you find yourself unable to go to sleep until early in the morning
- A magnesium/calcium supplement at bedtime
- Doxylamine (brand name Unisom for Sleep), an antihistamine: 25 mg at night
- 5 HTP (5-hydroxytryptophan): 100 to 400 mg at night
- Dr. Jacob Teitelbaum's herbal Revitalizing Sleep Formula combination

Prescription sleep aids may also be appropriate for debilitating fatigue. These can include

- *Tricyclic antidepressants:* antidepressants can help with pain relief and with increasing serotonin levels, both functions that can facilitate improved sleep. Frequently prescribed for sleep disturbances are low-dose tricyclic antidepressants, including doxepin (brand names Adapin and Sinequan), amitriptyline (brand names Elavil, Etrafon, Limbitrol, and Triavil), desipramine (brand name Norpramin), and nortriptyline (brand name Pamelor). These drugs may provide long-term benefit for improving sleep.

- *Other antidepressants:* other antidepressants that may be prescribed include sertraline (brand name Zoloft), venlafaxine (brand name Effexor), fluvoxamine (brand name Luvox), fluoxetine (brand name Prozac) paroxetine (brand name Paxil), and mirtazapine (brand name Remeron). Typically, it can take six weeks before an antidepressant has any impact on sleep.

- *Trazodone (brand name Desyrel):* trazodone is a frequently prescribed antidepressant for sleep problems, aiding with stage 3 and 4 sleep. It's particularly helpful for those who wake up every hour, or wake up and then can't fall back to sleep.

- *Antianxiety/muscle relaxants/benzodiazepines:* these are drugs that can help improve sleep, relax muscles, and modulate brain and brain receptor sensitivity. The most frequently recommended drug is clonazepam (brand name Klonopin), a long-acting benzodiazepine. Others are lorazepam (brand name Ativan) and alprazolam (brand name Xanax). Habit-forming potential may be a concern with these drugs.

- *Hypnotics:* the hypnotic drugs include zolpidem (brand name Ambien), triazolam (brand name Halcion), temazepam (brand name

Restoril), flurazepam (brand name Dalmane), quazepam (brand name Doral), and estazolam (brand name ProSom). Habit-forming potential may be a concern with these drugs. The drug zaleplon (brand name Sonata) is considered non-habit forming and may be a better option than the potentially habit-forming hypnotics.

In addition to adequate sleep, if you are suffering from flagging energy, you need to be sure that you are getting enough B vitamins. Vitamin B_{12} in particular is essential for energy. To ensure you're getting enough B vitamins, consider taking a B complex, plus a separate sublingual B_{12}.

Other supplements useful for fighting fatigue are substances that the body naturally produces. Supplements in this category include coenzyme Q10, also known as CoQ10, which supplies energy to muscles; L-carnitine; NADH (the reduced form of nicotinamide adenine dinucleotide), which helps cells convert food into energy; and DHEA (dehydroepiandrosterone) (but be sure to be tested by your practitioner before you start this hormone).

Professor Gayle Greene, author of *Insomniac*, has found that menopause is a time when hormonal fluctuations can especially affect sleep. Says Greene:

> Menopause is a biological as well as psychosocial event, a time when our bodies are adjusting to plummeting levels of estrogen and progesterone. Researchers suspect it may be the fluctuations rather than the depletion of hormones that create the problems, because the other trouble spots for women's sleep are also times when hormonal levels fluctuate, not only at menarche and just before menstruation, when estrogen and progesterone levels drop, but just after a woman gives birth, when estrogen levels plummet from the high point they were at during pregnancy.
>
> One reason hormonal fluctuations disrupt sleep is that they raise temperature. Body temperature tends to decline as sleep comes on, so anything that keeps it elevated—an electric blanket,

a hot room, work or vigorous exercise too close to bedtime—may inhibit sleep. Anything that facilitates a drop in temperature, like a cool room or a hot bath, may bring on sleep. Hot flashes, of course, raise body temperature in a big way.

If sleep problems are a major concern, I highly recommend that you learn more by reading two terrific books: Gayle Greene's *Insomniac* and *Sleep, Interrupted,* by Dr. Steven Park. Both explore the critical role of sleep in health and have practical advice.

Weight Gain

Gynecologist and menopause expert Dr. Jan Shifren sums it up when she says, "To combat perimenopausal weight gain, you have to run to stay in place." The same can also be said for weight gain that occurs with an underactive thyroid.

One of the most essential steps for weight management is for every woman to start making the necessary dietary and exercise changes to minimize any extra weight gain right away, for example, by their late thirties, or as soon as they have a thyroid disease diagnosis.

I talked about the importance of exercise and some healthy nutritional changes that women can make in perimenopause/menopause, but what do you do if you're gaining weight or finding weight loss more difficult? Remember that you're not lazy or lacking willpower, so don't beat up on yourself. Your body is changing and not working the way it used to, and it does have to do with your hormones. When the thyroid is underactive, the metabolism can become so efficient at storing every calorie that even the most rigorous diet and exercise programs may not seem to work. Add in the hormonal changes of menopause, and things slow down even more. Your friend or spouse could go on the same diet as you, lose a pound or two—or even more—a week, and you might stay the same, or even gain weight, despite working just as hard.

Unfortunately, the combination of thyroid and menopause is a double whammy for women, and you may find that nothing you're doing will move the scale. But there are some solutions.

EVALUATE YOUR MEDICATIONS

Take a look at medications you are taking. There are a number of drugs that promote weight gain. These include

- Steroid anti-inflammatories (prednisone)
- The antithyroid drug propylthiouracil (PTU)
- Lithium
- Estrogen and progesterone independently, together as the "pill," or together in hormone therapy
- Antidiabetic drugs, like insulin
- Various antidepressants, especially Prozac, Paxil, and Zoloft
- Mood-stabilizing and anticonvulsant drugs such as those given for bipolar disorder, including lithium, valproate (brand name Depakote), and carbamazepine (brand name Tegretol)
- Beta blockers
- Sedatives
- Tranquilizers

CHECK YOUR BLOOD SUGAR

Consider getting your blood sugar tested. At a minimum, you can get a glucose level from a home test kit, but preferably, get a fasting glucose test to evaluate whether your blood sugar is normal, high-normal, or elevated. In late 2003, the American Diabetes Association recommended that the fasting glucose range for defining prediabetes be changed, down from 110 mg/dL to 100 mg/dL, meaning that a value of 100 mg/dL or above would lead to a diagnosis of impaired fasting glucose/prediabetes/insulin resistance. If it is high-normal or elevated, this can in part contribute to your difficulty losing weight. It is also a sign that you are becoming insulin-resistant, are prediabetic, or already have type 2 diabetes. If your blood sugar level is elevated, you should discuss going on an antidiabetic medication such as metformin (brand name Glucophage). Metformin, along with diet and exercise, can help prevent the progression of insulin resistance or prediabetes to full type 2 diabetes.

CONSIDER AN ANTIDEPRESSANT

Even if you do not suffer from depression, you might find that you have greater success fighting a weight problem if your doctor tries you on a course of antidepressants. A number of people have written to report that their diet/exercise plan suddenly began to work after their doctor prescribed a short course of antidepressant medication, like Prozac, Welbutrin, Effexor, or Paxil. It's worth discussing with your doctor. Welbutrin, in particular, is thought to be helpful in curbing cravings and addictions, and is not as likely to cause weight gain, which can be a side effect with some antidepressants.

CONSIDER A LOW-GLYCEMIC DIET

An effective method to combat insulin resistance and the inability to properly process simple carbohydrates is eating a low-glycemic, carbohydrate-controlled, calorie-controlled, fairly low-fat diet. Low-glycemic foods are foods that do not rank high on the glycemic index, which assigns values to foods based on their effect on blood sugar levels.

High-glycemic foods are sugary, starchy substances, like those made with white flour (pasta, bread, and crackers), white rice, many cereals, desserts, and anything else with a high sugar content (drinks, jams and jellies, and snack foods, for instance). You may feel frustrated that there's nothing left to eat. But you need to rethink your eating habits, shifting to a diet of low-fat protein sources (like chicken, turkey, fish, leaner cuts of other meats, and low-fat dairy products) and nonstarchy, high-fiber vegetables and fruits, along with certain grains.

There are numerous books and Web resources that provide information on the glycemic index of foods and beverages that you can consult. Generally, avoid sugar in all forms and emphasize lean sources of protein, some good fat, nonstarchy vegetables, and limited fruit. When you do eat starches, be sure they're high fiber, and eat them only in limited quantities.

Researchers have found that thyroid disease and menopause are linked to increased cravings for starchy/sugary carbohydrates. This increased craving for and intake of carbohydrates appears to stem from various changes in brain chemistry and sympathetic nervous system activity. As you eliminate the "bad" carbohydrates from your body, you'll eventually find the cravings reduced.

EAT ENOUGH PROTEIN

Protein is needed to build muscle and to maintain energy, so your diet should include sufficient levels of protein. Ideally, include a portion of lean protein in every meal and snack, and never eat a carbohydrate, whether vegetable, fruit, or starch, without an accompanying protein, because it helps slow down the digestion of the carbohydrate as it converts to sugar.

GET ENOUGH GOOD FAT

Essential fatty acids cannot be produced in the body, so you must get them through diet or supplements. The key essential fatty acids are

- Omega-3/alpha-linolenic acid (ALA), eicosapentaenoic acid (EPA), docosahexaenoic acid (DHA): found in fresh fish from cold, deep waters (for example, mackerel, tuna, herring, flounder, sardines, salmon, rainbow trout, and bass), linseed oil, flaxseeds and flaxseed oil, black currant and pumpkin seeds, cod liver oil, shrimp, oysters, leafy greens, soybeans, walnuts, wheat germ, fresh sea vegetables, and fish oil. Usually, your body can convert ALA into EPA, then into DHA.

- **Omega-6/linoleic acid/gamma linolenic acid (GLA):** found in breast milk; sesame, safflower, cotton, and sunflower seeds and oil; corn and corn oil; soybeans; raw nuts; legumes; leafy greens; black currant seeds; evening primrose oil (EPO); borage oil; spirulina; and lecithin. Linoleic acid in omega-6 can be converted into GLA.

DRINK ENOUGH WATER

Hypothyroidism and menopause can both cause water retention and bloating. Because you feel or look bloated or swollen, you may not be drinking enough water. The body will hold onto even more water more fiercely when you cut back on your water intake. Not drinking at least 64 ounces of water a day is counterproductive, as it will worsen bloating and cause dehydration, which slows metabolism.

Hypothyroidism also slows digestion and elimination, which can impede weight loss. Optimize digestion by making sure you get high levels of fiber every day. If you need help with regular elimination, consider adding a natural supplement, such as ayurvedic triphala, to aid in regularity.

GET ENOUGH FIBER

Fiber is essential to digestion and optimizing your weight loss efforts. It has minimal calories but can fill you up by adding bulk, and when consumed with carbohydrates, it helps modulate the insulin response and normalize blood sugar. There is a fair amount of scientific support for fiber's ability to increase your feeling of fullness after you eat and reduce your hunger levels. One study found that adding 14 grams of fiber per day was associated with a 10 percent decrease in calorie intake and resulted in weight loss of five pounds over four months. To add fiber, eat more raw vegetables and fruits; they have more fiber than cooked or canned. Limit cereals and breads to high-fiber only. Two slices of high-bran bread, for example, has 7 grams of fiber, compared with only 2 grams of fiber for white bread. Other good sources of fiber are nuts, beans, apples, oranges, broccoli, cauliflower, berries, pears, brussels sprouts, lettuce, prunes, carrots, and yams. Women up to age fifty need 25 grams of fiber per day; those over fifty should get at least 21 grams. If you can't get all your fiber from food, consider a fiber supplement.

Important warning: If you switch from a low-fiber to a high-fiber diet, be sure to take your thyroid medication at least an hour before eating breakfast, so absorption is not impaired. High-fiber diets can change dosage requirements, so six to eight weeks after starting a high-fiber diet, you may wish to have your thyroid function tested to be sure you don't need a dosage change.

KEEP TRACK OF WHAT YOU EAT

Studies have shown that people who write down everything they eat lose weight, even if they're not formally dieting, simply because the act of writing makes you more aware of your consumption and likelier to make better choices. Get a journal or use your cell phone, your BlackBerry, a notepad, your computer, a calendar, or a loose-leaf binder to record what you eat on a daily basis. It doesn't matter what form your record takes; it's the action of sitting down and thinking about your goals, what you're going to eat, and assessing what you've eaten that will make the difference.

If you want a more formalized way to keep close track of your nutritional intake and want a supportive community to help you follow your chosen approach, check out tools such as South Beach Diet Online, Ediets, Weight Watchers Online, and Calorie Count, all of which have detailed food-tracking programs, as well as online support communities and forums where you can share information and encouragement with others.

ESPECIALLY FOR PEOPLE WITH HYPOTHYROIDISM

No matter which plan you choose, when you are following a weight loss program, there are some particular considerations you need to keep in mind that apply specifically to you as someone with hypothyroidism.

Don't expect to lose weight quickly. Celebrate your resounding success if you lose even a pound a week. Do *not* compare your results with anyone else. And *don't* diet with a friend, unless she or he is hypothyroid too, because you're bound to feel frustrated if you compare your rate of loss to others.

You *have* to exercise. It's not optional. Weight-bearing/muscle-building exercise is critical to raising metabolism, and aerobic exercise helps burn calories. Even if you join a weight loss center that says you can lose weight without exercise, it's not likely to be true for you.

If you add fiber to your diet, have your thyroid function retested about six to eight weeks after you stabilize at your new level of fiber intake. You may need a change in your dosage of thyroid hormone replacement.

If you lose more than 10 percent of your body weight, it's time to get retested to see if you need to adjust your dosage of thyroid medication.

Many thyroid patients report that only when they dramatically cut down on starchy carbohydrates and sugars—eliminating things like bread, sugar, pasta, sodas, and desserts—and limiting carbs mainly to vegetables, with some fruit, are they able to lose weight. While there are thyroid patients who process carbs with no difficulty and can lose weight on a more old-fashioned food pyramid diet that emphasizes cereals, grains, and bread, they seem to be the exception rather than the rule.

Hopping on a scale to keep track of weight loss is important, but not as important as keeping track of measurements. Particularly for thyroid patients, who may have more early results in building muscle than in losing pounds, keeping track of measurements can provide important feedback and may even provide incentive on those days when you don't see much movement on the scale.

MY OWN PROGRAM

Many women thyroid patients who are trying to lose weight turn to my book *The Thyroid Diet* for help. That book outlines in great detail how to optimize your thyroid treatment so you stop gaining, or at least get in the right state of mind to lose weight. Then you learn what actually needs to be done to start losing. As many of us have learned the hard way, if your thyroid is not being fully and effectively treated, even the best diet and exercise program in the world won't work. Maximizing thyroid treatment, balancing hormones and the endocrine system, increasing a slow metabolism, and determining what to eat to lose weight are all covered in *The Thyroid Diet*.

I've rarely met a woman in her forties or older who has success losing weight on high-carb approaches, myself included. Nor have I found that many thyroid patients do well on an "all you can eat," steak-and-bacon, low-carb diet that has no calorie or fat restrictions. (Doesn't work for me!) In *The Thyroid Diet*, I recommend a low-glycemic (low-sugar) diet that limits carbohydrates overall, emphasizes "good" carbs (vegetables primarily), but with calorie and fat limits, and this is the kind of diet I follow.

If you need a detailed, structured, ongoing program, with weeks of extensive menus and recipes, I also recommend *The South Beach Diet*, which has an updated version that's known as *The South Beach Diet Supercharged*. It's a healthy diet based on eating the right carbs and right fats, and it's not difficult to follow. In addition to the book, there is a Web site and online membership program for *South Beach* that's not hard to follow and works well for thyroid patients.

As for exercise, I'm a huge fan of T-Tapp, which is discussed in Chapter 8. It works better for me than any other approach I've found.

In addition to my prescription thyroid medication, I'm taking several supplements to help with weight loss. There is no miracle diet supplement, but there are some supplements and herbs that *may* help in your weight loss efforts. I emphasize *may*, because there are no guarantees. Some supplements may do nothing at all for you; in fact, they may actually do the opposite (you'll be one of the few people who gain weight on something that's supposed to help!). Right now, I'm taking glucomannan before each meal. It's dietary fiber from the root of the konjac plant, and it comes in capsule form. It is believed to help in balancing blood sugar, lowering cholesterol, and creating a feeling of fullness. I know that it makes me feel full when I take it, so I can cut back on my intake. I'm also taking cinnamon with each meal. Cinnamon is thought to reduce blood sugar levels, increase natural production of insulin, and lower cholesterol levels. I also am using FucoThin, a supplement made of fucoxanthin, a derivative of brown seaweed that has reported fat-burning properties.

Some other supplements to consider are alpha lipoic acid, acetyl-L-carnitine, calcium, capsaicin/cayenne pepper, chromium picolinate, conjugated linoleic acid (CLA), glucosol, glutamine/L-glutamine, *Hoodia gordonii*, pantethine, pyruvate, taurine, vitamin C, and zinc. I have a detailed discussion of these supplements in my book *The Thyroid Diet*.

Finally, to stay on track, I rely on Dr. Steven Gurgevich's *Self-Hypnosis Diet*. You can get the book/CD version or the audiobook format, and both are terrific. For me, it's a great, relaxing, and very effective way to make sure that the desire to manage my weight translates into action—eating well, exercising, and taking care of myself. Pop in the CD, listen, and help shore up your motivation and desire to do the right thing.

Other issues that can interfere with your ability to lose weight are discussed in various places here and in *Living Well with Hypothyroidism*, as well as in greater depth in *The Thyroid Diet*. These include food allergies and sensitivities, candidiasis/yeast overgrowth, celiac disease/gluten (or wheat) sensitivity, parasites, the copper/zinc balance, adrenal imbalances, and estrogen and progesterone imbalances.

Depression/Anxiety

If your depression or anxiety is unrelieved by even your best efforts to treat the underlying hypothyroidism and hormonal imbalances, then it may need to be treated separately. This is not something to be embarrassed about; it's just an indication that your brain chemistry is interrelated with your endocrine system, and without balance in one, it's hard to become perfectly balanced in the other. Antidepressant treatments—such as conventional medications, herbal formulations, therapy, exercise, and support—can help balance the brain chemistry and relieve the depression or anxiety.

MEDICATIONS

Antidepressants are frequently prescribed as a treatment for depression/anxiety. They include mirtazapine (brand name Remeron), venlafaxine (brand name Effexor), nefazodone (brand name Serzone), and bupropion (brand name Wellbutrin); selective serotonin reuptake inhibitors (SSRIs), such as paroxetine (brand name Paxil), fluoxetine (brand name Prozac), and sertraline (brand name Zoloft); monoamine oxidase inhibitors (MAOIs), such as phenelzine (brand name Nardil) and tranylcypromine (brand name Parnate); and tricyclic antidepressants, such as sinequan (Adapin), amitriptyline (brand name Elavil), desipramine (brand name Norpramin), and impramine (brand name Tofranil). Your doctor will need to discuss the best option for you. If you are prescribed an antidepressant, it may take a few weeks, even a month or more, to start seeing the benefits. Don't give up after a week or two if you don't feel a difference. Remember that some antidepressants can become stronger or weaker in the presence of thyroid hormone, or can interfere with thyroid absorption, so discuss this with your doctor.

Medications to combat anxiety are sometimes prescribed for short periods of time. These include clonazepam (brand name Klonopin), lorazepam (brand name Ativan), and alprazolam (brand name Xanax). Buspirone (brand name Buspar) is a newer antianxiety medication that takes several weeks to become effective. In some anxiety disorders, beta blockers, such as propranolol (brand name Inderal), may also be helpful.

ALTERNATIVE SUPPLEMENTS

Since there are side effects associated with many antidepressants, some people try supplements. While St. John's wort (*Hypericum perforatum*) is often a popular choice, some experts believe that it can interfere with thyroid hormone replacement therapy, and so should be avoided. Other supplements used for depression include 5-hydroxytryptophan (5-HTP), an amino acid derivative and the immediate precursor to serotonin, a brain chemical responsible for feelings of well-being. Another supplement some find effective is tyrosine. Tyrosine is an amino acid used to create norepinephrine, a brain chemical that works as an appetite suppressant, stimulant, and antidepressant; many leading-edge researchers are proposing that depression stems directly from a deficiency of norepinephrine. Most people need two to three weeks in order to begin seeing some definite benefits.

Supplements that may help with anxiety include valerian extract, passion flower, and L-theanine. (Note: My favorite sleep aid, Jacob Teitelbaum's Revitalizing Sleep Formula, contains these ingredients. At lower doses, it can be used as a natural antianxiety supplement.)

OTHER APPROACHES

Other approaches that are helpful in addressing depression and anxiety are

- Therapy, which can be combined with medication
- Eating well and stabilizing blood sugar by avoiding sugary and starchy carbohydrates
- Including an essential fatty acid supplement
- Physical exercise and activity
- Getting some sunshine (especially during colder months) and vitamin D

Sexual Dysfunction

As many as 43 percent of women reportedly have some sort of sexual dysfunction, including low desire and/or pain during intercourse. Low sex drive is a common—but not often talked about—symptom of both hypothyroidism and perimenopause/menopause.

In a Red Hot Mamas survey of menopausal women,

- Seventy-five percent of the women surveyed reported having less sex since entering menopause.
- Sixty-eight percent reported experiencing pain during active sex.
- Fifty-one percent reported vaginal dryness.
- Seventy-nine percent of the women who had vaginal dryness said that it had an effect on their sex lives.

Low sex drive/sexual dysfunction is also a symptom that, unfortunately, does not get better over time, despite what doctors deem adequate treatment. Many people, women in particular, still complain of a lack of sexual desire even after their doctors consider the thyroid problem sufficiently treated or put them on hormone therapy.

If you suffer from sexual dysfunction, you need to be sure that you are getting optimal thyroid treatment. You may want to explore prescription hormone treatment, in particular, testosterone, which may help with libido.

Low sex drive may be a result of other health conditions. Diabetes and hypertension/high blood pressure can cause low sex drive in women. You should ask your doctor to discuss the diagnosable symptoms of depression with you, so you can assess whether or not you are depressed.

You should also discuss other prescription drugs you are taking, because some antidepressants, tranquilizers, and antihypertensives, as well as many illegal drugs such as cocaine and marijuana, can reduce sex drive. An estimated 40 percent of patients on antidepressants

report problems with sexual function, in particular, tricyclic antidepressants like clomipramine (brand name Anafranil) and some
SSRIs, such as Prozac, Paxil, Zoloft, and Lexapro. If you are being
treated for depression, you may want to consider asking your doctor about bupropion (brand name Wellbutrin), an antidepressant
not typically associated with sexual side effects.

Other drugs you'll want to discuss with your practitioner are

- Antihistamines like dephenhydramine (Benadryl), loratidine
  (Claritin), cimetidine (Tagamet), fixofenadine (Allegra), ranitidine
  (Zantac), and others
- Anticancer drugs: tamoxifen and raloxifene, used to prevent
  recurrent cancers
- Anticonvulsants: phenobarbital (brand names Luminal, Dilantin,
  Mysloine, and Tegretol)
- Antiandrogens: cimetidine and spironolactone
- Antihypertensives (blood pressure medications): including alpha
  blockers, beta blockers (brand names Inderal, Atenolol,
  and Tenormin), diuretics, and calcium channel blockers
- Antipsychotics: Thorazine, Haldol, and Zyprexa
- Antianxiety medications: Xanax and Valium
- Birth control pills
- Chemotherapy drugs

There is some evidence that appetite suppressants and opioid
pain drugs contribute to sexual dysfunction.

Exercise improves blood flow to all body parts. Research has
found that people who exercise regularly have higher levels of desire, greater sexual confidence and frequency, and an enhanced
ability to be aroused and achieve orgasm, no matter what their age.
The best type of exercise is aerobic exercise, because it can trigger
the release of endorphins, chemicals in the brain that create a feeling of well-being.

An important thing that you can do to help sexual dysfunction is to lose weight. Excess weight can affect your self-image, making you feel less sexy and less interested in sex. And, medically, being overweight can reduce libido. Some experts believe that a ten- to twenty-pound weight loss in an overweight woman reduces enough body fat to in turn substantially reduce levels of sex hormone–binding globulin (SHBG), which then unbinds (frees up) estrogen and testosterone, allowing them to get back to their regular functions in the reproductive system.

When there are other psychological and self-esteem issues preventing healthy sexual desire, therapy can sometimes help. Traditional psychotherapy may help identify and resolve root causes of problems, improve self-esteem, and teach new skills in self-expression. Communications or couples counseling may help improve the relationship. Sex therapy may help resolve specific dysfunctions and teach techniques that aid in sexual desire and satisfaction.

The prescription drug Viagra has been used with women, but it's not clear whether it can be used to treat sexual dysfunction. For women, more research is needed on prescription drugs that will help with sexual desire.

Some herbal and natural supplements are considered helpful for low sex drive. But supplements can have various—and sometimes serious—side effects, so you shouldn't self-treat. Talk to your practitioner regarding these products. Some supplements that may help with libido are

- **Arginine:** an amino acid
- **Asian ginseng (Panax ginseng):** can help increase sexual energy
- **Avena sativa/oat extract:** this supplement (main brand is Vigorex) reportedly does help with sex drive.
- **Damiana:** an herbal aphrodisiac from Mexico
- **Horny goat weed:** used by Chinese medicine herbalists to

improve sexual functions

- **Maca:** South American Royal Maca may help women with libido problems.
- **Zinc:** low levels of zinc have been associated with low sex drive in women.

In terms of lifestyle issues, you may need to schedule sex regularly with your partner, and be sure to take time for your relationship. Some practitioners suggest reading erotic literature or using a vibrator.

Menstrual Irregularities

Many women in perimenopause experience a variety of menstrual problems. Erratic, unpredictable periods are a hallmark of the perimenopausal period. But another menstrual issue, menorrhagia (extremely heavy periods), is also a problem for some women during perimenopause.

According to Dr. Jerilynn Prior, scientific director of the Centre for Menstrual Cycle and Ovulation Research in Vancouver, Canada, in perimenopause, approximately 25 percent of women have at least one episode of heavy flow, which usually occurs when cycles are regular and before the onset of skipped cycles. What constitutes a "heavy flow," or menorrhagia? Says Dr. Prior:

> Flow of more than 80 mL (almost 3 ounces) per menstrual period is considered menorrhagia.

Since most of us aren't measuring, how can you tell if you're having menorrhagia? According to Dr. Prior:

> Each soaked normal-sized pad or tampon holds approximately 5 mL of blood. To calculate the approximate amount of blood loss, multiply the number of soaked normal-sized pads or tam-

pons in a whole cycle by five to determine the millilitres of blood lost. A maxi-tampon or pad probably holds 10 mL. Sixteen soaked normal-sized sanitary products used in one flow means a blood loss of 80 mL.

In comparison, during a normal period, a woman will typically soak two to seven sanitary products.

Hormone therapy—in particular, going on an oral contraceptive ("the pill")—can significantly improve menorrhagia. But what other options are there for women who do not want to take hormones?

First, there are some self-care measures. According to Dr. Prior:

> Any time you feel dizzy or your heart pounds when you get up from lying down it is evidence that the amount of blood volume in your system is too low. To help that, drink more and increase the salty fluids you drink, such as tomato or other vegetable juices or salty broths (like bouillon). You will likely need at least four to six cups (1.0–1.5 litres) of extra liquid that day. Take at least one tablet (200 mg) of ibuprofen every four to six hours. Nonsteroidal anti-inflammatories decrease the amount of flow by 25–30% by altering the endometrial prostaglandin balance. Also, start taking one tablet of over-the-counter iron (like 35 mg of ferrous gluconate) a day.

(Note: If you are also on thyroid hormone replacement, be sure that you are taking iron at least three to four hours apart from your thyroid medication.)

Some women have found that progesterone can be helpful. You can talk to your doctor about oral or transdermal prescription progesterone (the over-the-counter creams are usually not strong enough to affect heavy periods). Another option is the Mirena intrauterine contraceptive (from Bayer HealthCare Pharmaceuticals), which releases a synthetic progestin and can reportedly reduce total menstrual flow by as much as 94 percent.

There are some procedures that may help with heavy bleeding:

- Removing an intrauterine device (IUD) can help reduce menstrual flow.
- Operative hysteroscopy, in which a tiny tube known as a hysteroscope is inserted into the uterus, to view the uterine cavity and to visualize and surgically remove polyps that may be causing heavy menstrual bleeding
- Endometrial ablation, which uses ultrasound to permanently destroy the endometrium (the uterine lining) and may reduce menstrual flow significantly
- Endometrial resection, which involves using an electrosurgical technique to remove the uterine lining, which can also reduce heavy menstrual bleeding
- Hysterectomy, which removes the uterus, completely eliminating menstrual periods, but usually causing immediate surgical menopause

On the herbal and natural front, a number of plants have traditionally been used for heavy menstruation, including

- Royal Maca
- Red raspberry leaf tea (this is different from raspberry tea)
- Chasteberry/vitex
- Black cohosh
- Cramp bark tea or supplements
- Yarrow
- Nettles
- Shepherd's purse
- Marsh mallow

If you are a smoker experiencing menstrual problems, you have to stop smoking. Smoking is linked to many problems, including longer and heavier bleeding. The more you smoke, the more likely you are to have more significant symptoms. Find what works, whether it's antianxiety medication, antidepressants, varenicline (brand name Chantix), acupuncture, the nicotine patch, or a smoking cessation group, supplemented by exercise, stress reduction techniques, online support groups, and other tactics.

Hair Loss

During menopause, and for women with thyroid issues, the most common type of hair loss is androgenetic alopecia, also known as female pattern hair loss. Androgenic alopecia is affected by sex hormones (estrogen and progesterone), as well as by thyroid, adrenal, pituitary, and pineal hormones.

In androgenic alopecia, testosterone, a type of androgen hormone, is involved. Testosterone metabolizes to dihydrotestosterone (DHT), which causes hair follicles to react by interrupting the hair growth cycle and reducing follicle size. This causes changes in hair texture, diameter, and length.

Androgenic alopecia is characterized by a shortening of the hair's growth cycle and progressive shortening and thinning of individual hair shafts. It may progress until no hair growth is evident. It is most common in women around menopause. It's estimated that 37 percent of women experience hair loss and thinning around this time.

Hair can be considered a barometer of health because hair cells are some of the fastest growing in the body. When the body is in crisis, the hair cells can shut down to redirect energy elsewhere. Besides hormonal changes, poor diet and nutritional deficiencies, a variety of medications, surgery, and many medical conditions, noticeably, thyroid disease, can cause hair loss.

Many people notice rapid hair loss as a symptom of hypothyroidism. Some people feel this is the worst symptom of their thyroid problem: thinning hair, large amounts falling out in the shower or sink, often accompanied by changes in the hair's texture, making it dry, coarse, or easily tangled. Interestingly, some people have actually written to tell me that their thyroid problem was initially "diagnosed" by their hairdresser, who noticed the change.

Proper thyroid treatment, as well as estrogen and progesterone therapy, can help some cases of hormonally driven hair loss. If you're experiencing hair loss and are just starting hormone therapy, it's likely that the loss will slow down, and eventually stop, once hormone levels are stabilized and in the normal range. This may take a few months, however. Rest assured, I've had many thousands of e-mails from people and have yet to hear from anyone who lost all his or her hair, or became bald, due to hormone imbalances. But many people—including myself—have experienced significant loss of hair volume. In my case, I'd guess at one point I had lost almost half my hair. I had long, thick hair, and it got much thinner for a while.

If you continue to lose hair, you need to make sure that it's not caused by your particular type of thyroid hormone replacement. Prolonged or excessive hair loss is a side effect of Synthroid and other brands of levothyroxine in some patients. Many doctors do not know this, even though it is a stated side effect in the patient literature, so don't be surprised if your doctor is not aware of this.

When I have had major bouts of hair loss (despite low-normal TSH and being on a T4/T3 drug), I took the advice of several noted thyroid experts. In his book *Solved: The Riddle of Illness*, Stephen Langer, MD, points to the fact that symptoms of essential fatty acid insufficiency are very similar to hypothyroidism. Langer recommends evening primrose oil, an excellent source of essential fatty acids, for people with hypothyroidism. The usefulness of EPO, particularly in dealing with excess hair loss associated with hypothyroidism, was reinforced by endocrinologist Kenneth Blanchard. According to Dr. Blanchard:

> For hair loss, I routinely recommend multiple vitamins, especially evening primrose oil. If there's any sex pattern to it—if a woman is losing hair in partly a male pattern—then the problem

is there is excessive conversion of testosterone to dihydrotestosterone at the level of the hair follicle. Evening primrose oil is an inhibitor of that conversion. So almost anybody with hair loss probably will benefit from evening primrose oil.

As someone who has had a few periods of extensive hair loss since I became hypothyroid, I can vouch for the fact that after taking EPO, not only did my hair loss slow down, but it stopped after about two months. New hair grew back, and my hair was no longer straw-like, dry, and easily knotted. Now as soon as I notice my hair starting to shed, I start taking EPO again, usually 500 mg, two to three times a day.

If you have extensive or continued hair loss, you should consult with a dermatologist for more intensive treatment. Some of the key treatments are

- *Corticosteroids:* "steroid" drugs, usually injected into the patchy spots affected by alopecia, taken orally or administered topically as an ointment or cream

- *Finasteride (brand name Propecia):* the drug finasteride is available by prescription only as an oral treatment approved by the U.S. Food and Drug Administration (FDA) for androgenic alopecia. Finasteride decreases the level of DHT circulating in the blood. It is not approved for use by women of child-bearing age due to the highly increased possibility of fetal birth defects in women using or handling the pills. Some studies have found that finasteride use in postmenopausal women may be safe and can work as well or better than minoxidil.

Without a prescription, you can try minoxidil (brand name Rogaine). This drug, which comes in a topical solution, may slow down hair loss. In some people, it helps trigger hair regrowth after several months. Minoxidil is an FDA-approved remedy for hair loss.

The LaserMax laser comb is the only FDA-approved consumer device to treat hair loss. It's expensive, usually around $500, and the results are mixed. You might want to try several laser treatments at a salon to see if your hair loss responds before considering purchasing a LaserMax.

In addition to EPO, some other natural approaches that are helpful for hair loss are

- B vitamins
- DHEA
- Green tea
- Iron
- Lysine
- L-arginine
- Methylsulfonylmethane (MSM)
- Saw palmetto
- Pygeum/beta sitosterol
- Zinc
- Nettles

Also, be sure that you are not taking a medication that is a known trigger for hair loss. My book *The Thyroid Guide to Hair Loss* has detailed information on thyroid-related hair loss, prescription, natural, and mind–body approaches, and a detailed list of medications that cause hair loss.

Vaginal Dryness, Urinary/Bladder Symptoms

Vaginal dryness can be a side effect of lower estrogen levels in perimenopause and menopause. Oral and topical estrogen tends to resolve this symptom. In women who choose not to take hormones or use any of the natural herbal approaches to hormone balancing, there are some other options to help with vaginal dryness.

Vaginal moisturizers such as Replens and KY Long Lasting Vaginal Moisturizer can be applied periodically to help maintain moisture in the vaginal area and keep the cells lining the vagina moist. This may help relieve symptoms such as itching and a tendency toward irritation and infection. For sufficient lubrication during sexual intercourse, water-based vaginal lubricants like KY Personal Lubricant and Astroglide may be helpful.

You may also want to avoid antihistamines, as they have a tendency to dry out the mucous membranes, including the vagina.

Some practitioners also recommend Kegel exercises and regular sex to help tone pelvic muscles and improve blood supply to the pelvic area.

Urinary problems, including chronic infections, can be more common in menopause. To help prevent urinary infections, you'll want to urinate both before and after sexual intercourse, don't let your bladder remain full for long periods of time, and stay well hydrated. You'll want to limit alcohol, and be aware that smoking can aggravate bladder infections.

For incontinence, Kegel exercises have been shown to be more effective than many medications.

To perform Kegels, first identify the muscle groups by trying to stop your urine stream while you're urinating. These are the muscles used in Kegel exercises. Contract these muscles as tightly as you can, count to ten, then relax. You'll want to do ten contractions a day, three times a day, for maximum benefit. Experts suggest you do Kegels while you're waiting in line, in the car, at a store, or at your desk. For an extra challenge, try coughing or laughing while practicing.

Sex educator Kim Switnicki has developed a special DVD, *The Freedom from Your Leaky Bladder Program*, which helps teach proper Kegels and other techniques specifically to treat urinary incontinence. It's an excellent instructional guide.

For difficult urinary incontinence, talk to your doctor about medical options that can include

- Medications, including oxybutynin (brand names Dirtopan and Oxytrol), tolterodine (brand name Detrol), darifenacin (brand name Enablex), folifenacin (brand name Vesicare), and trospium (brand name Sanctura), that can help calm an overactive bladder
- Electrical stimulation devices that run pain-free mild electrical current into the bladder area to strengthen the muscles
- Collagen implants in the urethra
- Surgery to help prevent pelvic sagging

Hot Flashes/Night Sweats

Practitioners, from the most conventional to the most holistic, admit that if you are suffering from hot flashes and night sweats, the most effective treatment is some form of estrogen therapy. Studies show that estrogen therapy stops hot flashes and night sweats in 80 percent of patients and reduces their frequency and severity in the rest of women. You can't argue with those sorts of results.

At the same time, there are some very real issues regarding the safety of estrogen. Some women suffering from hot flashes and night sweats may, based on their own medical history or risk factors or based on concerns about the potential dangers of treatment, choose not to pursue this treatment. In those cases, the value of symptom relief is not worth the potential risks of the medication.

Some phytoestrogens, for example, flaxseed, soy, and black cohosh, may be worth investigating. But again, effectiveness is mixed, and we don't know if long-term use of phytoestrogens is safe.

Let's take a look at some other options for hot flashes, besides estrogen treatment.

OTHER MEDICATIONS

Although only hormones are approved by the FDA for treating hot flashes and night sweats, but doctors can prescribe other medications (called off-label prescriptions) for such use. Off-label prescriptions may be covered by some health insurance programs.

The most effective appears to be the antidepressants venlafaxine (brand name Effexor) and paroxetine (brand name Paxil), which, in some studies, have reduced hot flashes by as much as 61 percent at a daily dose of 150 mg. Side effects include dry mouth, loss of appetite, nausea, constipation/diarrhea, headache, dizziness, insomnia, and sexual dysfunction. At higher doses, these medications can raise blood pressure, so they are not recommended for women with hypertension. The FDA requires that all antidepressants carry a generic warning about possible suicide risk for patients taking them. Other antidepressants, including fluoxetine (brand name Prozac) and citalopram (brand name Celexa), have not been found to be effective for hot flashes and night sweats.

Gabapentin (Neurontin) is a medication approved for treating seizures as well as pain associated with shingles. One study found that 900 mg of gabapentin per day for twelve weeks resulted in a 46 percent decrease in hot flashes. Some women have found that a dose of gabapentin at night can help with night sweats. Side effects can include drowsiness, dizziness, nausea, imbalance when walking, and swelling.

Clonidine (brand name Catapres) is a high blood pressure medication. Transdermal use of a clonidine patch may help relieve hot flashes and could be useful for women who have high blood pressure and are not candidates for venlafaxine. Side effects include dizziness, drowsiness, dry mouth, low blood pressure, constipation, and inhibition of orgasm in women.

PRACTICAL CHANGES

Figure out if you have hot flash triggers. Some women have hot flashes like clockwork if they are drinking alcohol, have too much caffeine, or eat spicy food. Try keeping a "hot flash diary" for a few weeks, to learn your triggers, so that you can avoid them during this period of hormonal transition.

There's nothing worse than wearing a heavy wool sweater that you can't take off when a hot flash hits. So dress in layers, so that you can add or subtract clothing items as needed, and try to wear breathable cotton as much as possible.

Try to manage the ambient temperature as much as possible. This may mean turning down the thermostat to keep your home or office cooler during the day. Definitely keep temperatures cooler at night for sleeping. Some women like to have windows open or fans running.

It may seem silly, but a personal fan can really help. For summer heat, there are small portable fans that also have a water-misting feature. You can pop out a small battery-operated purse fan anywhere you need it, to help get through a several-minute hot flash more comfortably.

Some women like to keep ice water handy at all times. Carry a sports bottle or travel cup with ice water everywhere you go, and if you feel a hot flash coming on, sipping the ice water may help. You can even freeze a water bottle to keep in your car, or at the office, and as it thaws, you'll have a ready supply of ice water available.

Your fitness and weight can have an impact on hot flashes, so continuing to exercise may help regulate the nervous system and help with hot flashes. Also, helping reduce the frequency and severity of hot flashes is yet another benefit of losing weight and quitting smoking.

PACED RESPIRATION AND BREATHING

Gynecologist and menopause expert Dr. Jerilynn Prior recommends doing anything that decreases your feeling of stress as a way to help night sweats and hot flashes. In particular, she recommends paced breathing and guided visualization.

Good evidence supports what is called "paced breathing." It is a kind of meditation or relaxation therapy that uses slow, deep, controlled breathing. Alternate methods of relaxation are to sit in the same quiet place and relaxed way and visualize yourself in the most calm, secure, and lovely place you can imagine.

A study showed that paced respiration, when done twice daily, actually decreased the frequency of hot flashes by 50 percent over a four-month period. Other studies of paced respiration have shown that women who practice it also have lower average skin temperature, which is a way of measuring hot flashes.

Paced respiration is not hard, but it takes some practice. It's a diaphragmatic breathing technique, which means you need to keep your rib cage still and inhale and exhale using your stomach muscles to lower and raise your diaphragm. You can try it yourself.

- Start by sitting in a comfortable, quiet place.
- Inhale for five seconds, deeply into the abdomen and try not to move your rib cage.
- Exhale for five seconds, pulling your stomach muscles in and up.
- Repeat this cycle of breathing.

To practice, spend ten to fifteen minutes twice a day. When you feel a hot flash coming on, stop whatever you are doing, find a quiet place, and perform paced respiration until the hot flash subsides. You may even be able to prevent the hot flash from developing. A few minutes of paced respiration can also help calm stress during a hectic day.

Another form of breathing that may help for hot flashes is a yoga technique known as alternate nostril breathing. Alternate nostril breathing is thought to provide balance to the body's temperature, and some women swear by it as a hot flash remedy. To perform alternate nostril breathing,

- Sit on the floor in the lotus position, with legs comfortably crossed, or on a couch or chair, making sure your spine and head are aligned.
- Rest your left hand on your left knee or in the lap.
- With your right hand, place your index and middle finger at the center of your eyebrows.

- Keep the left nostril open and close the right nostril with the thumb of your right hand.
- Inhale slowly and deeply to the count of four, hold the breath for a count of two, then exhale through the left nostril to the count of four.
- Keeping your index and middle finger on your forehead between the eyebrows, release the thumb from the right nostril, and use the ring/fourth finger of the right hand to close the left nostril.
- Keep the right nostril open. Inhale slowly and deeply to the count of four, hold the breath for a count of two, then exhale through the right nostril to the count of four.

That is one cycle of alternate nostril breathing. Repeat the cycle, starting with one to two minutes, and working up to several sessions of ten minutes a day.

You might also want to try alternate nostril breathing when you are getting a hot flash, to see if it helps reduce the severity, intensity, or length of the flash.

Finally, I have to share the approach created by holistic physician Molly Roberts. In her work with groups of perimenopausal and menopausal women, Dr. Roberts realized that most women tense up and become very stressed when they are having a hot flash. Many of her patients also described hot flashes as a problem, something to be cured, or evidence that something is "wrong" with them.

Dr. Roberts believes that, like labor pains in childbirth, hot flashes are not evidence of something wrong, or unnatural, but rather are a natural process. Says Roberts:

Our bodies are such a miracle, there must be some constructive reason for hot flashes. I believe, therefore, that at some point, we're going to find out that hot flashes are actually good for us! What I think is happening is that as estrogen goes up and down, we have more tendency for blood clots. I think the opening of blood vessels during a hot flash may be helping to open up the vessels and perhaps even prevent clots.

Dr. Roberts realized that aspects of the Bradley method, which focuses on relaxation and natural abdominal breathing during childbirth to manage pain, might be useful for women suffering hot flashes. She created a process she calls "The Roberts Method for Hot Flashes," which she describes here.

When you have a hot flash, take it as a cue that you may be experiencing some stress. Consider a hot flash your body's way of saying, "Chill out and take a break." At the same time, recognize that there's something protective about hot flashes—they are natural and you are having them for a reason. Take a minute or two to do some deep, diaphragmatic breathing, and appreciate your body, appreciate how your body is figuring it all out and getting you through this time.

Dr. Roberts suggested this method to a group of women participating in a menopause workshop, and they tried it for a few weeks. The group then came back together, and most of the women reported that it really made a great deal of difference in the number of hot flashes they were having, as well as the length of time the hot flashes lasted. Dr. Roberts was particularly surprised that some of the women came back saying that they had even come to enjoy their hot flashes. Apparently, the hot flash became a reminder—and, at the same time, permission—to take a few moments to relax and do the deep breathing, which the women found pleasurable.

SELF-HYPNOSIS

A 2008 article in the *Journal of Clinical Oncology* reported on the results of a study of hypnosis for hot flashes. The women in the study received five fifty-minute sessions each week that involved relaxation and cooling imagery. The group reported a phenomenal 68 percent reduction in the severity and frequency of hot flashes.

As discussed in the section on affirmations and self-hypnosis in Chapter 9, I recommend Dr. Steven Gurgevich's self-hypnosis resources for perimenopause/menopause, or work with a medical hypnotist who is certified by the American Society of Clinical Hypnosis.

A Special Note: Stop Smoking!

I know that those of you who smoke hear it all the time, but one of the best things you can do to help resolve many symptoms is to quit smoking. Smoking makes thyroid problems worse, it makes menopausal symptoms worse, it makes menstrual irregularities worse, and it can make fatigue worse—not to mention the issues of heart and lung health.

Stopping smoking should be an essential part of your wellness plan.

Even if you've tried to quit smoking many times, don't despair. Keep trying, because eventually, you'll get good at it. I know, because I smoked for fifteen years, and I was not a social smoker; I was a hard-core, one-to-two-pack-a-day smoker. I tried to quit many times, but I loved to smoke and kept lapsing. Finally, I was able to quit in my early thirties. The only way I was able to do it was with the support of my doctor, some medication, and discovering that crocheting, of all things, could occupy my hands and mind enough for me to battle the cravings. (Five king-size afghans and three months later, I was finally smoke free for good, and I've stayed that way for another fifteen years.) While quitting smoking was one of the hardest things I have ever done, it's also one of the best things I could do. Even while facing the health challenges of thyroid disease and perimenopause, I thankfully do not have the extra risk of heart disease, stroke, lung cancer, emphysema, and a host of other smoking-related problems hanging over me. So find what works for you—antidepressants, antianxiety medications, smoking cessation drugs like Chantix, prayer, meditation, exercise, yoga, breathing, needlework, biofeedback—and get started.

chapter 11

Creating
YOUR OWN PLAN

If you always do what interests you, at least one person is pleased.

—*Katharine Hepburn*

When you are putting together your plan for managing wellness in your forties, fifties, and beyond, there are a number of things to keep in mind as you move forward to make that plan effective and empowering.

Cover the Basics

First, let's start by outlining the basics. These are the items that every woman needs to include in her wellness plan.

RESOLVE THYROID HORMONE IMBALANCES

Get any thyroid imbalances properly diagnosed, sufficiently treated, and optimized. That may require traditional approaches with prescription medications, but more likely it will require a broader, more integrative approach. The best thyroid treatment is the one that safely resolves your symptoms. You shouldn't be afraid to work with a doctor who is willing to try different approaches and integrate holistic, natural, and alternative medicine into your overall thyroid treatment.

MANAGE REPRODUCTIVE HORMONE IMBALANCES

When reproductive hormonal imbalances are interfering with your quality of life, get them properly diagnosed and sufficiently treated. Because prescription hormones carry some risks, you may want to try natural, holistic, lifestyle, and mind–body approaches first, to see if you lessen the frequency and severity of symptoms, and learn new tools to effectively respond to them. But when symptoms are unmanageable, you should not be afraid to investigate the use of prescription hormones. Right now, the best approach is to go with the safest hormones, at the lowest dose, for the least amount of time needed to resolve symptoms. Which ones are safest is somewhat controversial, but there's enough evidence to suggest that, whenever possible, stay away from the conjugated estrogens and synthetic progestins, and instead choose estradiol and other bioidentical estrogens, ideally in transdermal rather than oral forms, and natural forms of progesterone if you still have your uterus.

ADOPT A HEALTHIER WAY OF EATING

We are increasingly coming to understand the essential role that diet plays in helping us stay healthy and in helping maintain hormone balance. Many dietary changes were already discussed in Chapter 7, and while we all wish we could pursue a perfect diet, that's unrealistic. But all of us can try to reduce portion sizes; eat more organic foods so that we can avoid pesticides and hormones; eat more vegetables, fruits, and fiber; eat less processed, sugary, and starchy foods; ensure that we get good fats in our diet and minimize unhealthy, saturated fats; drink enough water; limit alcohol; and learn how to eat to live and not live to eat. We can also commit to trying new foods and learning how to use certain foods as "natural medicine" to help us deal with various symptoms we are experiencing.

EXERCISE

If there is one thing I would suggest to every woman reading this book, it's to exercise. Chapter 8 talks about T-Tapp, walking, and various other approaches, but in the end, whatever you do, commit to doing it. Slow and steady wins the race, as they say, and they're right. It's less important what you choose to do; what is important is consistency and discipline to stick with it. I have a dear friend, Jane, who is in her forties, in perimenopause, and I have watched in amazement as Jane has discovered the wonders of walking. She gets out there every morning, rain or shine, and walks briskly around her neighborhood. Her only fitness equipment is a pair of sneakers and her resolve to walk. In about eight months, Jane, who is a phenomenal cook and still loves to eat, has walked off fifty pounds and walked herself right into a size 6. I have no doubt that it's her resolve to keep walking that has been the secret to her success.

GET ENOUGH SLEEP

If I told you there was something that you could do every day that would help you lose weight, feel great, have amazing energy, help balance hormones, and help you live a longer life (and, oh, it's so easy even a baby can do it), would you try it? Of course you would. So put getting enough sleep right up there on your priority list of things to do to take care of your health.

The body is meant to rest, and despite all the improvements of the twenty-first century, we still haven't figured out a way to bypass the need for sleep. That means, for most of us, eight hours a night. Yes, eight hours.

PRACTICE REGULAR STRESS REDUCTION

Just like brushing your teeth every day is part of good dental health, reducing your stress every day is part of good mental health. What you do to incorporate stress reduction into your life is up to you. Some people pray or go to religious services, others take yoga or tai chi classes; some like breathing exercises; some meditate; some practice self-hypnosis or guided imagery; some use biofeedback; some pursue creative projects. It doesn't matter which method you choose. Just be sure that you find what works for you, that you find an approach that allows your body and mind to enjoy the "relaxation response," and make it a habit to incorporate it into your daily life.

FIND THE RIGHT PRACTITIONER

Finding a doctor who can help you with hormonal balance is a challenge. But perimenopause/menopause is an important time in your life to have a doctor who has time for you and who is your partner.

There is no single medical specialty that thoroughly prepares doctors for diagnosing and managing women's hormones, including thyroid, during the perimenopausal/menopausal period. There are actually many different types of practitioners—including endocrinologists, general practice or family practice doctors, internists, ob-gyns, nurse practitioners, antiaging medicine practitioners, and osteopaths, to name a few—as well as holistic and integrative practitioners, including holistic MDs, naturopaths, herbal medicine experts, and traditional Chinese medicine practitioners, who end up working with women on managing hormones. How do you know which one to choose?

I've put together some guidelines and advice to help you find the right practitioner for you, and, once you have that person, how to best communicate with him or her.

Forget Endocrinologists

While endocrinologists have traditionally considered thyroid disease and hormones as areas within the purview of endocrinology, let's be honest here. Endocrinologists can be essential for proper diagnosis and treatment of serious diseases of the thyroid, such as thyroid cancer and life-threatening thyroid storm, as well as severe endocrine problems, including adrenal conditions like Cushing's disease and Addison's disease, osteoporosis, polycystic ovary syndrome, and other complicated endocrine conditions. Diabetes, when improperly managed, can cause blindness, loss of limbs, and even death, is on the rise in the United States. At the same time, there is a severe shortage of endocrinologists. Right now, there are an estimated 4,000 endocrinologists in the United States serving the 25 million to 100 million Americans who might reasonably need to be seen by such specialists. That's only one for every 6,250 to 25,000 people.

Given such a shortage, where do you think endocrinologists are going to focus their energy? On women who don't feel well because of hormone imbalances, Hashimoto's thyroiditis, and symptomatic estrogen/progesterone imbalances? Or on people who have life-threatening endocrine diseases? (I'm not suggesting that hormone imbalances aren't serious or worthy of attention, of course, just trying to help explain how endocrinologists view them.)

Increasingly, endocrinologists are leaving it to other physicians—general practitioners, internists, ob-gyns, and such—to diagnose and manage what they consider "routine" hormonal imbalances of the thyroid and reproductive hormones, because as far as they are concerned, these patients don't need the specialized knowledge of an endocrinologist anyway. The American Association of Clinical Endocrinologists (AACE) says that keeping the thyroid in balance requires only "three easy steps": testing thyroid-stimulating hormone (TSH), taking medication, and following up with a TSH test every six to twelve months.

My advice? Unless you have what an endocrinologist would view as a life-threatening endocrine disease, look elsewhere for assistance in diagnosing and managing thyroid and reproductive hormone imbalances.

If you have an endocrine disease, however, and need to find a qualified endocrinologist, the AACE maintains an online "Find an Endocrinologist" database of clinical endocrinologists, by state. The American Thyroid Association (ATA) also has a "Find a Thyroid Specialist" database featuring doctors who are members of the American Thyroid Association. The Endocrine Society's Hormone Foundation educational arm maintains a "Find an Endocrinologist" search function. My Thyroid Top Doctors database online also includes endocrinologists who are recommended by thyroid patients.

Consider a Certified NAMS Menopause Practitioner

The North American Menopause Society (NAMS) has a certification process for designation as an NAMS menopause practitioner. To receive this certification, a practitioner must pass a competency exam. The NAMS maintains a state-by-state list of practitioners who have received this certification, which is good for three years. The list includes MDs, osteopaths, naturopathic physicians, physician's assistants, nurse practitioners, pharmacists, nurses, clinical social workers, and psychologists. Some of the practitioners will clearly have a more conventional focus; the naturopathic and osteopathic physicians on the list may have a more holistic and integrative approach.

The NAMS recommends that you contact doctors in your area to find out what percentage of their practice is devoted to menopause. The NAMS then suggests that you schedule an appointment to see if the practitioner and the practice are a good fit for you.

Information on how to access the list of certified NAMS menopause practitioners is featured in Appendix A.

Use Other Referral Opportunities

There are a variety of referral services, most online, that provide additional starting points to help you identify conventional and integrative practitioners. These include

- American College of Obstetricians and Gynecologists
- American Society for Reproductive Medicine
- American Osteopathic Association
- American Holistic Health Association

Contact information for these groups and their referral services is featured in Appendix A.

New York Times health writer and advocate Tara Parker-Pope has other good advice. Says Parker-Pope:

> If you are lucky enough to know a nurse, [he or she] can be an excellent resource to help you find the best doctors.

Take an Integrative Approach

While many general practitioners and family practice doctors are called on to diagnose and treat thyroid disease or recognize and treat perimenopausal/menopausal symptoms, they are doing so without a great deal of knowledge or expertise about either issue.

You can't assume that the thyroid treatment or hormone advice you are getting from a general practitioner (GP) or family practice doctor is reflecting the best and most current thinking on the issue.

Many GPs and family doctors are not proactive about testing the thyroid in perimenopausal/menopausal women, and if they do, they only know how to order a TSH test. These doctors tend to rely on the laboratory report to flag abnormal results, which means that, because most labs are still using the old, outdated TSH range, they are usually not going to be aware that TSH levels above 2.5 to 3.0 may be indicative of thyroid problems.

Frequently, when it comes to what are considered classic menopausal symptoms (that is, hot flashes and night sweats), these doctors don't test hormones at all, but simply recommend Premarin or Prempro.

There are, of course, terrific doctors who follow a conventional approach. But if you're trying to find the right practitioner to partner with you for hormonal wellness, my advice is, if you can afford it, see a holistic/integrative practitioner who has experience working with hormone imbalances. By "holistic/integrative," I mean a practitioner who combines the best of conventional approaches with holistic, natural, and alternative medicine approaches and will help identify the best of all possible worlds for you in terms of your treatment.

The challenges are in how and where to find these practitioners and, given that few of them are covered by health insurance plans, paying for them.

Jacob Teitelbaum, MD, an expert on integrative medicine, says a more broad-minded practitioner is especially important for proper thyroid care:

> General doctors don't do thyroid—they *think* they do thyroid, but they don't know how to do it properly. If you want it properly done, go to a holistic physician.

To find qualified integrative physicians, Dr. Teitelbaum suggests starting with the American Board of Integrative Holistic Medicine (ABIHM). ABIHM maintains a physician locator service for more than 1,000 board-certified integrative and holistic doctors around the country. Contact information for ABIHM is in Appendix A.

I'm not suggesting that there are no GPs or family practice doctors who haven't made an effort to become especially knowledgeable about balancing hormones, because they are out there. But you will have to actively seek them out, either through referrals from their satisfied patients or through directories, such as my Thyroid Top Doctors Directory online.

Communicate Well with Your Doctor

One of the most essential things about communicating with your doctor is to interact professionally. Some women approach a doctor's appointment as if it were coffee with girlfriends. We go in and we complain: "I feel so fat, I feel like I just inhale chocolate, and I'm gaining weight," or "I am so totally exhausted," or "My husband's going to kill me; I just don't want sex," and so on. Doctors tend to hear an informal style of expressing our symptoms as more emotional than physical, which is why these sorts of complaints may be met with recommendations to take antidepressants rather than evaluated as possible thyroid or hormonal issues.

So when you meet with your doctor, be prepared to express your symptoms in a less emotional, more quantifiable way. Quantifying your symptoms is an important way to get doctors to really *hear* what you're saying about your concerns. So, for example, instead of saying, "I'm totally exhausted, I can't drag myself around," you can say, "I used to manage a busy life—forty-hour-a-week job, caring for an aging parent—on seven hours a night. Now I need nine hours a night, and I am still tired." Or, instead of saying, "Everything I eat is ending up on my hips!" say, "I was maintaining my weight on about 2,000 calories a day and going to the gym three times a week. Now I've actually stepped it up to five times a week, an hour each time, and dropped my calories down to 1,800 a day, and I'm still gaining approximately one pound a week."

Tara Parker-Pope sums it up this way:

> Women need to learn that the doctor visit is not catching up with an old friend. Think about how you'd talk to your accountant or mechanic. Your relationship with your doctor is special, and it shouldn't be cold, but beyond the warm feelings, you need to be very specific, and help your doctor by giving [him or her] the best information.

One of the most important things you can do to make your doctor's visits productive is to have an agenda. Some patients find it helpful to put together a simple list of key points to discuss with the doctor, in order of priority, and bring two copies to the appointment.

This helps ensure that all your key issues are covered and that you haven't left the most important questions for the end of the visit.

Another way to get the most out of your visit is to keep a health diary. Says Parker-Pope:

> When you start keeping track of things like sleep, events, foods, and symptoms, you start to see patterns. I think before you go to the doctor, you should keep a health diary for at least a few weeks or more. And don't just keep track of obvious symptoms; write down major things—thoughts, how you feel. Women are smart, we can see changes. And doctors respect health diaries; it takes the emotion out of a doctor's visit.

During the visit, take notes if necessary, or if you want to concentrate on what the doctor is saying, think about bringing a tape recorder with you. (Easy-to-operate digital audio recorders, which are the size of a cell phone, can record hours.)

Better yet, think about bringing a family member or friend to important doctor's visits. In fact, bringing a companion with you on a medical visit is associated with improved satisfaction and better communication. Your companion can help by taking notes, asking follow-up questions, and generally aiding in communication.

One of the key challenges in getting properly diagnosed and treated for thyroid and hormone imbalances is finding enough time. It takes time to explore symptoms and review medical history, and often there simply isn't enough time to cover everything during a regular visit.

Of course, holistic or integrative practitioners, most of whom are not on any insurance plans, often spend more time with their patients, as a hallmark of their care. But many of us cannot afford to go outside our insurance plan. If you are limited to seeing only certain practitioners, how can you get as much time as possible for your hormonal evaluation?

Tara Parker-Pope has an excellent idea: schedule an annual physical. Says Parker-Pope:

> Insurance and HMOs give you one annual physical, and that can be a longer appointment that gives you a lot more time with your doctor. During your physical, ask for a complete workup. Tell the doctor you'd like to look at your blood levels for thyroid, hormones, cholesterol, blood sugar, a complete blood count, and so on.

Some doctors debate the value of blood tests for hormones and don't use them, or they are trying to contain costs and will only test for thyroid hormone if faced with a patient who has serious symptoms. If the doctor refuses to test you or suggests that you start on hormones like estrogen without a test, Parker-Pope suggests that you tell the doctor you're willing to consider it, but that you'd like to rule out other issues first.

Stay Informed and Connected

Patient advocate and *Good Morning America* medical correspondent Marie Savard, MD, believes that being informed and connecting with others is essential.

> Be informed. . . . [I]t's important to understand your body and what to expect. Sometimes just understanding the physiologic changes can help more than other approaches . . . it puts your mind at ease. Don't hesitate to share your experience with friends and family who may have gone through the same thing.

> Follow the health news. Keep in mind that a lot of coverage of health in the media is sensationalized or oversimplified. In some cases, reporters simply don't understand what they're talking about.

Here are just a few of the sources I rely on for health news coverage related to thyroid disease and menopause:

- *New York Times* (including the Well Blog online, from Tara Parker-Pope, who is especially knowledgeable about hormones)
- Andrew Weil's Self-Healing newsletter, for alternative health information
- North American Menopause Society's monthly Menopause Flashes e-newsletter
- Google alerts, for the latest news articles published (I have it set to retrieve all new articles published on thyroid, menopause, and hormones, among other topics.)
- *Power-Surge Online* newsletter
- *Prevention* magazine

I also regularly access the latest medical research on thyroid disease, hormones, and other topics of interest through the National Library of Medicine's PubMed service online, at http://www.pubmed.gov.

If you're interested in thyroid disease, you'll also want to subscribe to my various newsletters on thyroid disease, including a weekly and monthly e-mail newsletter and my bimonthly print newsletter. Information on how to sign up is in Appendix A.

Stefanie Rotsaert, a thyroid patient and founder of a successful patient support group in New Jersey, has found that being informed and connecting with others are part of her overall wellness plan.

Before I had my second thyroid surgery, I was very frustrated. So I started reading everything, looking at alternatives, talking to doctors.

Later, after her surgery, Rotsaert noted in a hospital evaluation form that there were support groups for many issues in her area but not for thyroid disease. The next thing she knew, she was launching a support group through her hospital. The group, going strong for a number of years, is now independent. Through it, Rotsaert books various practitioners to speak to members, and members share information with each other.

Many local hospitals, YMCAs, and community organizations have support groups for women in menopause, so in-person support is always an option. Also, keep in mind that there are wonderful support forums on the Internet for menopause and thyroid disease. I'd encourage you to visit the friendly Minnie Pauz forum, Power-Surge, and my own thyroid forums, for information and support. Links are available online at www.menopausethyroid.com.

When You Don't Have Access to the Internet

When I speak with folks around the country during phone coaching sessions or in-person seminars, I frequently will suggest checking out this or that Web site. I'm always saying, "You can find that on the Internet at http://www . . . " but it's not uncommon for someone to respond, "But I don't have the Internet at home," or "I don't have a computer," or "I don't know the first thing about surfing the Web!"

Unfortunately, if you want to stay up on health information, it's a hardship these days if you don't have Internet access. There are entire categories of information that are difficult, or unwieldy, or down-right impossible to get any other way. There are many online support groups, e-mail newsletters, and Web-based organizations out there ready to meet many of your health care information needs. But these groups do not operate using 800 numbers and regular mail.

If you think there's no hope for you to get this information because you don't have access to the Internet, think again. Just head over to your local public library. According to the American Library Association:

Internet access in public libraries is as common as books. Almost all public library outlets offer public access to the Internet. For people without computers at home, work or school, libraries are the number one point of access to the Internet.

Your local librarians are trained to help you find what you need, including online.

Listen to Your Own Wisdom

Who should we listen to when it comes to menopause? Should it be our mothers? Our best friends? Our doctors? Oprah?

I asked many of the doctors I interviewed this question, and I have to say, Tieraona Low Dog's answer resonated with me. Dr. Low Dog said that, ultimately, we should listen to our own wisdom.

Who do we look to? We should look within. Don't look outside yourself for experts. When I'm in the quiet, I can hear my own inner wisdom . . . and that may help me to know how to proceed, and where to find the answer.

Dr. Low Dog then shared a compelling quote from Ralph Waldo Emerson, and I think it's fitting to end the book with it:

These are the voices which we hear in solitude, but they grow faint and inaudible as we enter into the world.

RESOURCES

This is an abbreviated list of key resources. A lengthy, detailed resources list, featuring recommended books, Web sites, and organizations to support you in your effort to live well, along with listings of menopause and hormone clinics around the United States, is featured online at http://www.menopausethyroid.com. The Web site also features detailed downloadable Risks/Symptoms Checklists for Thyroid Disease and Perimenopause/Menopause.

The Menopause Thyroid Solution

The Menopause Thyroid Solution
WEB SITE   http://www.menopausethyroid.com
Home page for this book, featuring detailed resources links and information, articles, newsletters, support groups, and more for women interested in integrative approaches to living well with thyroid disease, perimenopause, and menopause.

Mary Shomon's Health and Thyroid Web Sites

Mary Shomon's "Thyroid-Info" Web Site
WEB SITE   http://www.thyroid-info.com
The Internet's most popular thyroid patient Web site since 1997, featuring articles, forums, books, newsletters, and the latest news on all facets of thyroid disease.

Thyroid Top Doctors Directory
WEB SITE   http://www.thyroid-info.com/topdrs
A directory of patient-recommended top thyroid practitioners, from
around the country and the world, organized by state and country.

Thyroid Site at About.com
WEB SITE   http://thyroid.about.com
Managed by Mary Shomon since 1997, the Thyroid Site at About.com, part
of the New York Times Company, features hundreds of articles, links to top
sites on the Internet, a weekly newsletter, support community, and more.

Sticking Out Our Necks: The Thyroid Patient Newsletter

Sticking Out Our Necks is Mary Shomon's newsletter, designed to keep
thyroid patients up-to-date on important thyroid-related and health news,
both conventional and alternative. The twelve-page print newsletter is
published every other month, sent by mail; the e-mail news summary goes
out monthly online.

Sticking Out Our Necks Print Newsletter
WEB SITE   http://www.thyroid-info.com/subscribe.htm

Thyroid-Info
P.O. Box 565, Kensington, MD 20895-0565
TELEPHONE   888-810-9471
WEB SITE   http://www.thyroid-info.com/newsletters.htm
E-MAIL   news@thyroid-info.com

Mary Shomon's Books

*The Thyroid Hormone Breakthrough: Overcoming Sexual and
Hormonal Problems at Every Age.* HarperCollins, 2006
WEB SITE   http://www.thyroidbreakthrough.com
An integrative look at diagnosing and treating thyroid problems in
conjunction with all aspects of hormonal health, including puberty, PMS,
menstrual cycle, fertility, pregnancy, postpartum, breastfeeding, libido,
sexual function, and menopause.

Living Well with Hypothyroidism: What Your Doctor Doesn't Tell You . . .
That You Need to Know. HarperCollins, 2005
WEB SITE   http://www.thyroid-info.com/book.htm
This best-selling book, first published in 2000, updated/revised in a second
edition in 2005, features conventional and alternative information on
every aspect of hypothyroidism, from getting diagnosed, to treatment, to
alternatives, to residual symptoms such as fatigue and weight gain.
Special issues such as pregnancy, depression, and life after thyroid cancer
are explored.

Living Well with Graves' Disease and Hyperthyroidism: What Your
Doctor Doesn't Tell You . . . That You Need to Know. HarperCollins, 2005
WEB SITE   http://www.thyroid-info.com/graves
A comprehensive look at the conventional and alternative approaches to
Graves' disease and hyperthyroidism, including the first detailed protocol
for natural management of an overactive thyroid. Evaluates the pros and
cons of the key treatments, including antithyroid drugs, radioactive
iodine, surgery, and natural approaches. Explores nutritional approaches
and long-term management.

The Thyroid Diet: Manage Your Metabolism for Lasting Weight Loss.
HarperCollins, 2004
WEB SITE   http://www.GoodMetabolism.com
The first book to tackle the critical connection between weight gain and
thyroid disease, offering a conventional and alternative plan for lasting
weight loss. A *New York Times* and Amazon.com bestseller and a Quills
Award semifinalist, the book identifies the frustrating impediments to
weight loss for thyroid patients and offers solutions, both conventional
and alternative, to help. With food lists, menus, supplement
recommendations, handy worksheets to use in weight loss tracking, and a
special resource section featuring Web sites, books, and support groups.

Living Well with Autoimmune Disease: What Your Doctor Doesn't Tell
You . . . That You Need to Know. HarperCollins, 2002
WEB SITE   http://www.autoimmunebook.com
The definitive guide to understanding mysterious and often difficult-to-
pinpoint autoimmune disorders like thyroid disease, Hashimoto's
thyroiditis, Graves' disease, multiple sclerosis, rheumatoid arthritis,
Sjögren's syndrome, lupus, alopecia, irritable bowel syndrome, psoriasis,
Raynaud's syndrome, among others, and a road map to finding both

conventional and alternative diagnosis, treatment, recovery, and, in some cases, even prevention or cure.

Living Well with Chronic Fatigue Syndrome and Fibromyalgia: What Your Doctor Doesn't Tell You . . . That You Need to Know. HarperCollins, 2004
WEB SITE   http://www.cfsfibromyalgia.com
An integrative approach to diagnosis and treatment of chronic fatigue syndrome and fibromyalgia, two conditions that are more common in thyroid patients and that share similar symptoms. While most books promote one particular theory and treatment approach, *Living Well with Chronic Fatigue Syndrome and Fibromyalgia* looks at the bigger picture by exploring a myriad of theories and treatment options, from conventional therapies such as medication and vitamins to alternative approaches.

Other Recommended Books on Thyroid Disease

In addition to Mary Shomon's books on thyroid disease, the following books are recommended.

Arem, Ridha. *The Thyroid Solution: A Revolutionary Mind–Body Program for Regaining Your Emotional and Physical Health.*
Ballantine Books, 2007

Barnes, Broda Otto. *Hypothyroidism: The Unsuspected Illness.*
HarperCollins, 1976

Blanchard, Kenneth. *What Your Doctor May Not Tell You about Hypothyroidism.* Grand Central Publishing, 2004

Brownstein, David. *Iodine: Why You Need It, Why You Can't Live Without It.*
Medical Alternatives Press, 2008
WEB SITE   http://www.drbrownstein.com

Brownstein, David. *Overcoming Thyroid Disorders.*
Medical Alternatives Press, 2002
WEB SITE   http://www.drbrownstein.com

Friedman, Theodore C. *The Everything Health Guide To Thyroid Disease: Professional Advice on Getting the Right Diagnosis, Managing Your Symptoms, and Feeling Great.* Adams Media, 2006

Langer, Stephen, and James F. Scheer. *Solved: The Riddle of Illness.* McGraw-Hill, 2006

Moore, Elaine, and Lisa Moore. *Graves' Disease: A Practical Guide.* McFarland & Co., 2001
WEB SITE   http://www.elaine-moore.com/gravesdisease

Shames, Richard, and Karilee Shames. *Feeling Fat, Fuzzy or Frazzled?* Hudson Street Press, 2005
WEB SITE   http://feelingfff.com

Shames, Richard, and Karilee Shames. *Thyroid Power: Ten Steps to Total Health.* Collins Living, 2002
WEB SITE   http://www.thyroidpower.com

Teitelbaum, Jacob. *From Fatigued to Fantastic!* Avery, 2007
WEB SITE   http://www.endfatigue.com

Thyroid-related Web Sites and Support Forums

About.com Thyroid Forums
WEB SITE   http://forums.about.com/ab-thyroid

Alt.support.thyroid
WEB SITE   http://www.altsupportthyroid.org/

American Thyroid Association
WEB SITE   http://www.thyroid.org

Broda Barnes Research Foundation
WEB SITE   http://www.brodabarnes.org

Dr. David Brownstein's site
WEB SITE   http://www.drbrownstein.com

Dr. Jacob Teitelbaum's site
WEB SITE   http://www.endfatigue.com

Edna Kyrie's Thyroid Research
WEB SITE   http://www.thyroidresearch.com

Elaine Moore's Graves' and Autoimmune Disease Education site
WEB SITE   http://www.elaine-moore.com

Endocrineweb
WEB SITE   http://www.endocrineweb.com

Hormone Foundation
WEB SITE   http://www.hormone.org

Thyroid Disease Manager
WEB SITE   http://www.thyroidmanager.org

Thyroid Forums
WEB SITE   http://www.thyroid-info.com/forums

Thyroid Support listserv
WEB SITE   http://health.groups.yahoo.com/group/thyroid/

Thyroid and Autoimmune Patient Advocacy Groups

American Autoimmune Related Diseases Association
22100 Gratiot Avenue East, Detroit, MI 48021
TELEPHONE 586-776-3900   WEB SITE http://www.aarda.org

Broda Barnes Research Foundation
P.O. Box 110098, Trumbull, CT 06611   TELEPHONE 203-261-2101
FAX 203-261-3017   WEB SITE http://www.brodabarnes.org

Thyroid Drugs and Their Manufacturers

Tapazole, Levoxyl, and Cytomel
King Pharmaceuticals, Inc., 501 Fifth Street, Bristol, TN 37620
TELEPHONE 800-776-3637/423-989-8000   WEB SITE http://www.kingpharm.com

   Levoxyl   TELEPHONE 866-LEVOXYL (538-6995)
   WEB SITE http://www.levoxyl.com
   Cytomel   WEB SITE http://www.kingpharm.com/kingpharm/
   products/product_details.asp?id_product=36
   Tapazole   WEB SITE http://www.kingpharm.com/kingpharm/
   products/product_details.asp?id_product=47

Armour Thyroid, Thyrolar, and Levothroid
Forest Pharmaceuticals, Professional Affairs Department, 13600 Shoreline
Drive, St. Louis, MO 63045   TELEPHONE 800-678-1605, ext.7301
FAX 314-493-7457   WEB SITE http://www.forestpharm.com

> *Armour Thyroid* WEB SITE http://www.armourthyroid.com
> *Thyrolar* WEB SITE http://www.thyrolar.com
> *Levothroid* WEB SITE http://www.levothroid.com

Unithroid
Jerome Stevens Pharmaceuticals, distributed by Lannett Pharmaceuticals,
9000 State Road, Philadelphia, PA 19136
TELEPHONE 800-325-9994/215-333-9000

Westhroid/Nature-Throid
Western Research Laboratories, 2404 West 12th Street, Suite 4, Tempe,
AZ 85281   TELEPHONE 877-797-7997/623-879-8537   FAX 623-879-8683
WEB SITE http://www.westernresearchlaboratories.com

> *Nature-Throid* WEB SITE http://www.nature-throid.com/
> *Westhroid* WEB SITE http://www.wes-throid.com/

Synthroid
Abbott Laboratories, 100 Abbott Park Rd., Abbott Park, IL 60064-3500
TELEPHONE 800-255-5162
WEB SITE http://abbott.com, http://www.synthroid.com

Thyrogen
Genzyme Therapeutics, 500 Kendall Street, Cambridge, MA 02142
TELEPHONE 800-745-4447/617-768-9000   WEB SITE http://www.thyrogen.com

Perimenopause/Menopause Books and Guides

Here are some recommended books about menopause. More detailed descriptions of the books are available online at http://www.menopausethyroid.com.

Adams, Dee. *Laugh Your Way through Menopause with "Minnie Pauz."*
Lulu Press, 2007   WEB SITE http://www.lulu.com/content/965290

Brownstein, David. *The Miracle of Natural Hormones.* Medical
Alternatives Press, 2006   WEB SITE http://www.drbrownstein.com

Clark, Carolyn Chambers. *Living Well with Menopause: What Your Doctor Doesn't Tell You . . . That You Need to Know*. HarperCollins, 2005
WEB SITE http://www.carolynchambersclark.com/

Early Menopause Guidebook (6th ed.). North American Menopause Society, 2006 WEB SITE https://store.menopause.org

Gittleman, Ann Louise. *Before the Change: Taking Charge of Your Perimenopause*. HarperSanFrancisco, 2004
WEB SITE http://www.annlouise.com

Kantrowitz, Barbara, and Pat Wingert Kelly. *Is It Hot in Here? Or Is It Me? The Complete Guide to Menopause*. Workman Publishing, 2006

Lee, John R., and Virginia Hopkins. *What Your Doctor May Not Tell You about Menopause: The Breakthrough Book on Natural Hormone Balance* (rev. ed). Time Warner Book Group, 2004
WEB SITE http://www.johnleemd.com/store/more_menopause.html

Menopause Guidebook (6th ed.). North American Menopause Society, 2006
WEB SITE https://store.menopause.org

Menopause Practice: A Clinician's Guide (3rd ed.). North American Menopause Society, 2007 WEB SITE https://store.menopause.org

Parker-Pope, Tara. *The Hormone Decision*, Rodale Books, 2007

Reiss, Uzzi, and Yfat Reiss Gendell. *The Natural Superwoman: The Scientifically Backed Program for Feeling Great, Looking Younger, and Enjoying Amazing Energy at Any Age*. Avery, 2007
WEB SITE http://www.uzzireissmd.com

Reiss, Uzzi, and Martin Zucker. *Natural Hormone Balance for Women: Look Younger, Feel Stronger, and Live Life with Exuberance*. Atria, 2002

Perimenopause/Menopause Web Sites and Support Forums

HysterSisters WEB SITE http://go.to/hystersisters

Menopause at About.com WEB SITE http://menopause.about.com

Minnie Pauz, with Dee Adams   WEB SITE http://www.minniepauz.com

Minnie Pauz Forum   WEB SITE http://www.minniepauz.com/forum

North American Menopause Society   WEB SITE http://www.menopause.org/

Power-Surge   WEB SITE http://www.power-surge.com/

Power-Surge Forum   WEB SITE http://www.power-surge.com/php/forums

Rebecca Hulem, The Menopause Expert
WEB SITE http://www.themenopauseexpert.com/

Red Hot Mamas   WEB SITE http://www.redhotmamas.org

Women's Health at About.com   WEB SITE http://womenshealth.about.com

Key Perimenopause/Menopause Advocacy Groups

American Association of Clinical Endocrinologists
1000 Riverside Avenue, Suite 205, Jacksonville, Florida 32204
TELEPHONE 904-353-7878   WEB SITE http://www.aace.com

American Menopause Foundation, Inc.
350 Fifth Avenue, Suite 2822, New York, NY 10119
TELEPHONE 212-714-2398   WEB SITE http://www.americanmenopause.org

The Centre for Menstrual Cycle and Ovulation Research (CeMCOR)
The Gordon and Leslie Diamond Health Care Centre, 2775 Laurel Street,
Room 4111, Vancouver, BC V5Z 1M9
TELEPHONE 604-875-5927   FAX 604-875-5915
WEB SITE   http://www.cemcor.ubc.ca/

North American Menopause Society
P.O. Box 94527, Cleveland, OH 44101   TELEPHONE 440-442-7550
FAX 440-442-2660   WEB SITE http://www.menopause.org

Testing

Bellevue Pharmacy
1034 South Brentwood Boulevard, Suite 102, St. Louis, MO 63117
TELEPHONE 800-728-0288/314-727-8787   FAX 800-458-9182/314-727-2830
WEB SITE http://www.bpharmacysolutions.com/hormone/lab.asp

The Canary Club
WEB SITE http://www.canaryclub.org

Diagnos-Techs, Inc.
Clinical and Research Laboratory, 6620 South 192nd Place, Building J,
Kent, WA 98032 TELEPHONE 800-878-3787
WEB SITE http://www.diagnostechs.com

Genova Diagnostics (formerly Great Smokies Diagnostic Laboratory)
63 Zillicoa Street, Asheville, NC 28801 TELEPHONE 800-522-4762/828-253-0621 WEB SITE http://www.genovadiagnostics.com

MyMedLab
TELEPHONE   888-MYMEDLAB (888-696-3352)
WEB SITE http://www.thyroid-info.com/mymedlab

Tissue Mineral Analysis Testing
Uni Key Health Systems, Inc., with Dr. Ann Louise Gittleman,
181 West Commerce Drive, P.O. Box 2287, Hayden Lake, ID 83835
TELEPHONE 800-888-4353; service: 208-762-6833 FAX 208-762-9395
WEB SITES   http://www.annlouise.com, http://www.unikeyhealth.com

Urinary Iodine Clearance Test/Hakala Research
885 Parfet Street, Suite E, Lakewood, CO 80215
TELEPHONE 877-238-1779/303-763-6242 WEB SITE http://www.hakalalabs.com

ZRT Laboratory
1815 N.W. 169th Place, Suite 5050, Beaverton, OR 97006
TELEPHONE 503-466-2445 FAX 503-466-1636
HORMONE HOTLINE 503-466-9166 WEB SITE http://www.salivatest.com

Estrogen/Progesterone Hormone Drugs and Their Manufacturers

Premarin, Prempro, Premphase, Enjuvia, Alora
Wyeth Pharmaceuticals, P.O. Box 8299, Philadelphia, PA 19101-8299
TELEPHONE   800-934-5556 WEB SITE http://www.wyeth.com

  Premarin WEB SITE http://www.premarin.com

  Prempro WEB SITE http://www.prempro.com

  Premphase WEB SITE http://www.premphase.com

Enjuvia   WEB SITE   http://www.enjuvia.com

Alora   TELEPHONE   888-ALORA4U   WEB SITE   http://www.alora.com

Climara/ClimaraPro/Menostar/Mirena/Angeliq
Bayer Health Care Pharmaceuticals; P.O. Box 1000, Montville, NJ 07045
TELEPHONE   888-84-BAYER (888-842-2937)
WEB SITE   http://pharma.bayer.com

Climara   WEB SITE   http://www.clearlyclimara.com

ClimaraPro   WEB SITE   http://www.climarapro.com

Menostar   WEB SITE   http://www.menostar-us.com

Mirena   WEB SITE   http://www.mirena-us.com

Angeliq   WEB SITE   http://www.angeliq-us.com

Vivelle-Dot/CombiPatch
Novartis Pharmaceuticals Corporation, One Health Plaza, East Hanover,
NJ 07936-1080   TELEPHONE   888-NOW-NOVA (888-669-6682)

VivelleDot   WEB SITE   http://www.vivelledot.com

CombiPatch   WEB SITE   http://www.combipatch.com

EstroGel, Prochieve
Ascend Therapeutics, 607 Herndon Parkway, Suite 210, Herndon, VA 20170
TELEPHONE   877-204-1013

Estrogel   WEB SITE   http://www.estrogel.com

Prochieve   WEB SITE   http://www.prochieve.com

Elestrin
PharmaDerm, 210 Park Avenue, Florham Park, NJ 07932
TELEPHONE   973-514-4240   FAX   973-514-4363
WEB SITE   http://www.pharmaderm.com   TELEPHONE   866-DERM-HLP
(866-337-6457)   WEB SITE   http://www.elestrin.com

Divigel
TELEPHONE   800-654-2299   WEB SITE   http://www.divigelus.com

Estrasorb
340 Martin Luther King Jr. Boulevard, Suite 500, Bristol, TN 37620
TELEPHONE   800-328-0255, 423-274-2100   FAX   423-274-2199
WEB SITE   http://www.estrasorb.com

Evamist
Ther-Rx Corporation, 1 Corporate Woods Drive, Bridgeton, MO 63044
TELEPHONE 314-646-3700, 877-567-7676
WEB SITE http://www.evamist.com

Estring
WEB SITE http://www.estring.com

Femring, FemHRT, Estrace, Femtrace
Warner Chilcott Pharmaceuticals; 100 Enterprise Drive, Rockaway, NJ 07866
TELEPHONE 973-442-3200 WEB SITE http://www.wcrx.com/index.php

   Femring WEB SITE http://www.wcrx.com/products/femring/index.php

   FemHRT WEB SITE http://www.wcrx.com/products/femhrt/index.php

   Estrace WEB SITE http://www.wcrx.com/pdfs/pi/pi_estrace_wc_imprint.pdf

   Femtrace WEB SITE http://www.wcrx.com/products/femtrace/index.php

Vagifem, Activella Novo Nordisk Inc., 100 College Road West, Princeton,
NJ 08540 TELEPHONE 609-987-5800, 866-668-6336
WEB SITE www.novonordisk.com

   Vagifem WEB SITE http://www.vagifem.com

   Activella WEB SITE http://www.activella.com

Provera
Pfizer Pharmaceuticals, 235 East 42nd Street, New York, NY 10017
TELEPHONE 866-706-2400/212-733-2323
WEB SITES http://www.pfizer.com,
          http://www.pfizer.com/products/rx/rx_product_provera.jsp

Prometrium
Solvay Pharmaceuticals, 901 Sawyer Road, Marietta, Georgia
30602 TELEPHONE 800-241-1643, ext. 8
WEB SITE http://www.prometrium.com

Estratest/Estratest HS
Solvay Pharmaceuticals, 901 Sawyer Road, Marietta, Georgia 30602
TELEPHONE 770-578-9000
WEB SITE http://www.solvaypharmaceuticals-us.com/products/
estratestmainprodpage/

Finding Doctors and Practitioners, Verifying Credentials

American Academy of Osteopathy
3500 DePauw Boulevard, Suite 1080, Indianapolis, IN 46268
TELEPHONE 317-879-1881
WEB SITE Find a Physician:
http://www.academyofosteopathy.org/findphys.cfm

American Association of Clinical Endocrinologists Database
WEB SITE http://www.aace.com/memsearch.php

American Board of Integrative Holistic Medicine
614 Daniel Drive NE, East Wenachee, WA 98802-4036
TELEPHONE 509-886-3046
WEB SITE http://www.holisticboard.org/D/locate_physician.html

American College of Obstetricians and Gynecologists Physician Finder
WEB SITE http://www.acog.org/member-lookup/disclaimer.cfm

American Holistic Health Association Referrals
P.O. Box 17400, Anaheim, CA 92817-7400 TELEPHONE 714-779-6152
WEB SITE http://ahha.org/referrals.asp

American Holistic Medical Association Doctor Finder
12101 Menaul Boulevard NE, Suite C, Albuquerque, NM 87112
TELEPHONE 505-292-7788 WEB SITE http://www.holisticmedicine.org

American Osteopathic Association
142 East Ontario Street, Chicago, IL 60611 TELEPHONE 800-621-1773/312-
202-8000 FAX 312-202-8200 WEB SITE http://www.aoa-net.org

American Society for Reproductive Medicine
WEB SITE http://www.asrm.org/search/providersearch.html

American Thyroid Association's Find a Thyroid Specialist Database
WEB SITE http://www.thyroid.org/patients/specialists.php3

Armour Thyroid/Thyrolar—Find a Prescribing Physician Database
WEB SITE http://www.armourthyroid.com/locate.html

The Cranial Academy
8202 Clearvista Parkway, #9-D, Indianapolis, IN 46256
TELEPHONE   317-594-0411/317-594-9299   WEB SITE Find a Professional:
http://www.cranialacademy.com/agreement.html

Credentialed NAMS Menopause Practitioners
WEB SITE   http://www.menopause.org/MPlist.pdf

Hormone Foundation Endocrinologist Database
WEB SITE   http://www.hormone.org/FindAnEndo/index.cfm

Mary Shomon's Thyroid Top Doctors Directory
WEB SITE   http://www.thyroid-info.com/topdrs

North American Menopause Society U.S. Practitioners
WEB SITE   http://www.menopause.org/cliniciansus.pdf

Compounding Pharmacies

Belmar Pharmacy
12860 West Cedar Drive, Suite 210, Lakewood, CO 80228
TELEPHONE 800-525-9473/303-763-5533   FAX 866-415-2923/303-763-9712
WEB SITE   http://www.belmarpharmacy.com

Knowles Apothecary/Brookville Pharmacy
10400 Connecticut Avenue, Suite 100, Kensington, MD 20895
TELEPHONE   301-942-7979   FAX 301-942-5544
WEB SITE   http://www.brookvillepharmacy.com

Women's International Pharmacy
12012 North 111th Avenue, Youngtown, AZ 85363;
2 Marsh Court Madison, WI 53718
TELEPHONE   800-279-5708   FAX 800-279-8011
WEB SITE   http://www.womensinternational.com

Herbs, Supplements, and Vitamins

Iherb.com (online only)
WEB SITE   http://www.iherb.com

Life Extension Foundation
WEB SITE   http://www.lef.org

Royal Maca/Whole World Botanicals:
P.O. Box 322074, Fort Washington Station, New York NY 10032
TELEPHONE   888-757-6026/212-781-6026
WEB SITE   http://www.wholeworldbotanicals.com

Willner (catalog, phone, in person)
100 Park Avenue, New York, NY 10017; 253 Broadway, New York, NY 10007;
2900 Peachtree Road NE, Atlanta, GA 30305
TELEPHONE 800-633-1106/212-682-2817   WEB SITE http://www.willner.com

Melatonin

International Anti-Aging Systems
A U.K.-based offshore pharmacy that carries Dr. Walter Pierpaoli's
specialized TI-MElatonin formulation, along with various vitamins and
supplements.
TELEPHONE   Order Hotline/U.S.: 866-800-4677 (toll-free from U.S.);
general inquiries/U.S.: 415-992-5563; outside U.S.: 44-208-123-2106/in U.K.:
(0208) 123-2106   WEB SITE http://www.antiaging-systems.com

Walter Pierpaoli, MD/Melatonin Research
WEB SITE   http://www.drpierpaoli.com

Pierpaoli, Walter (ed.). *Reversal of Aging: Resetting the Pineal Clock:
Annals of the New York Academy of Sciences.* Wiley-Blackwell, 2006

Pierpaoli, Walter, and William Regelson. *The Melatonin Miracle:
Nature's Age-Reversing, Disease-Fighting, Sex-Enhancing Hormone.*
Pocket Books, 1996

T-Tapp Exercises

Free video clips and instructions for a number of popular T-Tapp exercises
can be found at the T-Tapp Web site, http://www.t-tapp.com. T-Tapp offers
a variety of products to help meet fitness and exercise goals, including
Teresa Tapp's book with DVD, *Fit and Fabulous in 15 Minutes* (the "secret
to a flat stomach exercise" in the bonus DVD is especially popular with
women in perimenopause), and a number of DVD-based exercise videos,
including

- *Mindful Movement for Menopause Management*

- *T-Tapp Total Workout*

- *T-Tapp More Rehabilitative Program* (for people with more pounds to lose, more physical limitations, or more "candles on the cake")

- *Sit Down T-Tapp* (a T-Tapp workout done in a chair) and *T-Tapp Broom* (a T-Tapp workout done using a broom for balance and support)

The T-Tapp book is also available at Amazon.com, Barnes & Noble, and local bookstores.
TELEPHONE 800-342-0717/727-724-0123   WEB SITE http://www.t-tapp.com

Self-Hypnosis and Biofeedback

Gurgevich, Steven. *Self-Hypnosis for Perimenopause/Menopause.* Tranceformation Works, Behavioral Medicine, Ltd., 5215 North Sabino Canyon Road, Tucson, AZ 85750-6435
TELEPHONE 866-506-1700   WEB SITE http://www.tranceformation.com

Gurgevich, Steven, and Joy Gurgevich. *The Self-Hypnosis Diet: Use the Power of Your Mind to Make Any Diet Work for You Audio CD.* Sounds True WEB SITE http://www.tranceformation.com

Healing Rhythms Biofeedback Program, from Dr. Andrew Weil, Dr. Deepak Chopra, and Dr. Dean Ornish. The Wild Divine Project, P.O. Box 381, Eldorado Springs, CO 80025   TELEPHONE 866-594-WILD (9453)/303-499-3680   TELEPHONE 303-499-3688   WEB SITE http://www.wilddivine.com

Meditation and Breathing

These meditation and breathing resources are each available as a book and audio CD from in-person and online booksellers including Amazon.com and Soundstrue.com and as a downloadable audio from Audible, located at http://www.Audible.com

Breathing: The Masterkey to Self Healing/Meditation for Optimum Health (Audio CD)—Andrew Weil, MD, Sounds True, 2001

Meditation for Beginners: Six Guided Meditations for Insight, Inner Clarity, and Cultivating a Compassionate Heart—Jack Kornfield

WEB SITE   http://www.jackkornfield.org

WEB SITE   http://store.soundstrue.com/kornfieldj.html

How to Meditate, with Pema Chodron

WEB SITE   http://www.shambhala.org/teachers/pema/

WEB SITE   http://store.soundstrue.com/chodronp.html

Meditation in a New York Minute—Mark Thornton

WEB SITE   http://www.yescalm.org/

WEB SITE   http://store.soundstrue.com/thorntonm.html

Nutrition and Fitness Resources

Agatston, Arthur. *The South Beach Diet Supercharged: Faster Weight Loss and Better Health for Life.* Rodale Books, 2008
WEB SITE   http://www.SouthBeachDiet.com

Colbin, Annemarie. *The Book of Whole Meals: A Seasonal Guide to Assembling Balanced Vegetarian Breakfasts, Lunches and Dinners.* Ballantine Books, 1985   WEB SITE   http://www.foodandhealing.com

Colbin, Annemarie. *Food and Healing.* Ballantine Books, 1986
WEB SITE   http://www.foodandhealing.com

Colbin, Annemarie. *Natural Gourmet.* Ballantine Books, 1991
WEB SITE   http://www.foodandhealing.com

Gittleman, Ann Louise. *The Fat Flush Plan.* McGraw-Hill, 2001
WEB SITE   http://www.annlouise.com

Gittleman, Ann Louise. *The Gut Flush Plan: The Breakthrough Cleansing Program to Rid Your Body of the Toxins That Make You Sick, Tired, and Bloated.* McGraw-Hill, 2008
WEB SITE   http://www.annlouise.com

Gittleman, Ann Louise. *Hot Times: How to Eat Well, Live Healthy, and Feel Sexy during the Change*. Avery, 2005
WEB SITE   http://www.annlouise.com

Joanie Greggains' Pacewalk CD
WEB SITE   http://greggainshealthmatrix.com

Svec, Carol, and Marie Savard. *Apples and Pears: The Body Shape Solution for Weight Loss and Wellness*. Atria Books, 2007
WEB SITE   http://www.drsavard.com

Other Resources

Colbin, Annemarie. *The Basics of Healthy Cooking Video*
WEB SITE   http://www.foodandhealing.com/video.htm

Switnicki, Kim. *Freedom from Your Leaky Bladder: Get Your Life Back!* DVD
TELEPHONE   888-475-2948   WEB SITE http://www.bladderfreedom.com

Park, Steven, MD. *Sleep, Interrupted*. Jodev Press, 2008
WEB SITE   http://www.sleepinterrupted.com

Greene, Gayle. *Insomniac*. University of California Press, 2008

Holistic CDs from Drs. Bruce and Molly Roberts of Lighthearted Medicine
TELEPHONE   520-327-9624
WEB SITE http://www.lightheartedmedicine.com/products.html

- *In the Now:* mindfulness meditation with Dr. Bruce Roberts: audio CD

- *Sounds of the Garden:* audio CD

- *The Treasures Within* guided imagery meditation with Dr. Molly Roberts: audio CD

appendix b
EXPERTS

The following is contact information for many of the experts who graciously agreed to contribute information and interviews for *The Menopause Thyroid Solution*.

DAVID BROWNSTEIN, MD. – The Center for Holistic Medicine, 5821 West Maple Road, Suite 192, West Bloomfield, MI 48322 TELEPHONE 248-851-1600   WEB SITE http://www.drbrownstein.com

ADRIENNE CLAMP, MD, DABMA. – The Asclepeion Center, 9834 Capitol View Avenue, Silver Spring, MD 20910   TELEPHONE 301-495-0933 WEB SITE http://adrienneclampmd.com

ANNEMARIE COLBIN, PHD. – Natural Gourmet Institute for Health and Culinary Arts, 48 West 21st Street, 2nd floor, New York, NY 10010 TELEPHONE 212-645-5170   WEB SITE http://www.naturalgourmetschool.com, http://www.foodandhealing.com

JOCELYNE EBERSTEIN, LAC, DOM. – 10780 Santa Monica Boulevard, #245, Los Angeles, CA 90025-7633   TELEPHONE 310-446-1968 WEB SITE http://www.thelivingwellusa.com

ANN LOUISE GITTLEMAN, PHD, CNS. – Uni Key Health Systems, 181 West Commerce Drive, P.O. Box 2287, Hayden Lake, ID 83835 TELEPHONE 800-888-4353   WEB SITE http://www.annlouise.com

STEPHEN GURGEVICH, PHD, AND JOY GURGEVICH. – Sabino Canyon
Integrative Medicine, LLC, 5215 North Sabino Canyon Road, Tucson, AZ
85750-6435   TELEPHONE 866-506-1700/520-886-1700
WEB SITE http://www.tranceformation.com

CHARLES HAKALA. – Hakala Research, 885 Parfet Street, Suite E,
Lakewood, CO 80215   TELEPHONE 877-238-1779/303-763-6242
WEB SITE http://www.hakalalabs.com

HARRIET HALL, MD. – Science-based Medicine Blog
WEB SITE http://www.sciencebasedmedicine.org; http://www.skepdoc.info

DONNA HURLOCK, MD. – 205 South Whiting Street, Suite 303,
Alexandria, VA 22304   TELEPHONE 703-823-1533
WEB SITE http://www.dhurlock.yourmd.com

IRMA JENNINGS. – Certified holistic nutritional counselor, AADP
TELEPHONE 917-405-5410
WEB SITE http://www.nourishmentwithirma.com

RISA KAGAN, MD, FACOG. – East Bay Physicians Medical Group; clinical
professor, Department Of Obstetrics/Gynecology, University of California
at San Francisco, 2915 Telegraph Avenue, #200, Berkeley, CA 94705
TELEPHONE 510-204-8190

SCOTT KWIATKOWSKI, DO. – 8701 Georgia Avenue, Suite 406,
Silver Spring, MO 20910   TELEPHONE 301-718-3696
WEB SITE http://www.dohealth.org

TIERAONA LOW DOG, MD. – Director of Education, Program in
Integrative Medicine; clinical assistant professor, Department of
Medicine, University of Arizona, P.O. Box 64141, Tucson, AZ 85728-4141
TELEPHONE 520-760-8969   WEB SITE http://www.drlowdog.com
Dr. Tieraona Low Dog's Online School of Herbal Medicine
WEB SITE http://www.botanicalmedicineinstitute.com

MARTIN MULDERS, MD. – 2505 Boulevard of the Generals, Jeffersonville,
PA 19403; 610-630-8600   WEB SITE http://drmulders.com

VIANA MULLER, PHD. – Whole World Botanicals, P.O. Box 322074 Fort Washington Station, New York NY 10032   TELEPHONE 888-757-6026/212-781-6026   WEB SITE http://www.wholeworldbotanicals.com

WALTER PIERPAOLI, MD. – Research director, Neuroimmunomodulation Laboratory at the Italian National Research Center on Aging; scientific director, Jean Choay Institute for Biomedical Research in Switzerland; president, Interbion Foundation for Basic Biomedical Research, Via San Gottardo 77, 6596 Gordola (TI), Switzerland
WEB SITE http://www.drpierpaoli.com

JERILYNN PRIOR, MD, FRCPC. – The Centre for Menstrual Cycle and Ovulation Research, The Gordon and Leslie Diamond Health Care Centre, Room 4111, 2775 Laurel Street, Vancouver, BC Canada V5Z 1M9
TELEPHONE 604-875-5927   WEB SITE http://www.cemcor.ubc.ca/

UZZI REISS, MD. – 414 Camden Drive, Suite H, Beverly Hills, CA 90210
TELEPHONE 310-247-1300   WEB SITE http://www.uzzireissmd.com

TERI ROBERT, PHD. – Help for Headaches and Migraine, P.O. Box 1726, Parkersburg, WV 26102-1726   WEB SITES http://www.helpforheadaches.com, http://www.healthcentral.com/migraine

MOLLY ROBERTS, MD. – LightHearted Medicine, 1701 East Lind Road, Tucson, AZ 85719   TELEPHONE 520-327-9624
WEB SITE http://www.LightHeartedMedicine.com

MARIE SAVARD, MD. – Author, patient advocate, ABC *Good Morning America* medical correspondent   WEB SITE http://www.drsavard.com

RICHARD SHAMES, MD, AND KARILEE SHAMES, RN, PHD. – P.O. Box 2466, Sebastopol. CA 95473
WEB SITES http://www.thyroidpower.com, http://www.feelingfff.com

JAN SHIFREN, MD – Associate professor, obstetrics, gynecology, and reproductive biology, Harvard Medical School; director, Vincent Menopause Program, Massachusetts General Hospital, 55 Fruit Street, Yawkee 10, Boston, MA 02114   TELEPHONE 617-726-8868

KIM SWITNICKI, ACC, ECPC. – Bladder Freedom, 201 Station A, Nanaimo, BC V9R 5K9 Canada   TELEPHONE 888-475-2948/250-753-8692 WEB SITE http://www.bladderfreedom.com

TERESA TAPP. – T-Tapp, 1450 10th Street South, Safety Harbor, FL 34695 TELEPHONE 800-342-0717/727-724-0123   WEB SITE http://www.t-tapp.com

JACOB TEITELBAUM, MD. – WEB SITE http://www.endfatigue.com

Agatston, Arthur, and Joseph Signorile. *The South Beach Diet Supercharged: Faster Weight Loss and Bett*er Health for Life. Rodale Books. 2008.

American Academy of Orthopaedic Surgeons. "Boomers: Tips on How to Exercise Safely." Press release, August 8, 2008.

American Association of Clinical Endocrinologists Web site, http://www.aace.com.

American Chemical Society. "Revealing Estrogen's Secret Role in Obesity." Press release, August 13, 2007.

Anderson D., et al. "Menopause in Australia and Japan: Effects of Country of Residence on Menopausal Status and Menopausal Symptoms." *Climacteric* 2004; 7(2):165–174.

Anderson, G. L., Limacher M., Assaf A. R., et al. (2004). "Effects of Conjugated Equine Estrogen in Postmenopausal Women with Hysterectomy: the Women's Health Initiative Randomized Controlled Trial." *Journal of the American Medical Association*, 291(14):1701–12.

Arafah, Baha. "Increased Need or Thyroxine in Women with Hypothyroidism during Estrogen Therapy." New England Journal of Medicine 2001 (June 7):1743–1749.

Arendt, Josephine. "Safety of Melatonin in Long-Term Use." *Journal of Biological Rhythms* 1997; 12(6):673–681.

Arthur, J.R. "Selenium and Iodine Deficiencies and Selenoprotein Function." *Biomedicine and Environmental Science*. 1997 Sep; 10(2-3):129–35.

Avis, N. E., et al. "Is There a Menopausal Syndrome? Menopausal Status and Symptoms across Racial/Ethnic Groups." *Social Science and Medicine* 2001; 52(3):345–356.

Bachmann, Gloria A. "Strategies for Recognition and Management of Sexual Dysfunction in Menopausal Women." *Medscape.* 2004. http://www.medscape.com/viewarticle/482219_2.

Balfe, P., et al. "Estrogen Receptors and Breast Cancer." *European Journal of Surgical Oncology,* 30(10):1043–1050.

Ballard, Karen, et al. "Beyond the Mask: Women's Experiences of Public and Private Ageing during Midlife and Their Use of Age-resisting Activities." *Health* 2005; 9(2):169–187.

Benvenga, S., et al. "Altered Intestinal Absorption of L-Thyroxine Caused by Coffee." *Thyroid.* 2008 Mar; 18(3):293–301.

Bogani, P., et al. "*Lepidium meyenii* (Maca) Does Not Exert Direct Androgenic Activities." *Journal of Ethnopharmacology.* 2006; 104(3):415–417.

Bohnet, H. G., et al. "Subclinical Hypothyroidism and Infertility." *Lancet* 1981; 2:1278.

Bromberger, J. T., et al. "Psychologic Distress and Natural Menopause: A Multiethnic Community Study." *American Journal of Public Health* 2001; 91(9):1435–1442.

Brownstein, David. *Iodine: Why You Need It, Why You Can't Live without It* (3rd ed.). Medical Alternatives Press. 2008.

Brownstein, David. *The Miracle of Natural Hormones.* Medical Alternatives Press. 2006.

Brownstein, David. *Overcoming Thyroid Disorders.* Medical Alternatives Press. 2002.

Butt, Debra A., et al. "Gabapentin for the Treatment of Menopausal Hot Flashes: A Randomized Controlled Trial." *Menopause* 2008; 15(2):310–318.

Cagnacci, A., et al. "Season of Birth Influences the Timing of Menopause." *Human Reproduction.* 2005 Aug; 20(8):2190–3.

Casper, Robert, et al. "Menopausal Hot Flashes." *Up to Date in Endocrinology and Diabetes* 2006 (September).

Ceccarelli, Claudia, and Walter Bencivelli. "[131]I Therapy for Differentiated Thyroid Cancer Leads to an Earlier Onset of Menopause: Results of a Retrospective Study." *Journal of Clinical Endocrinology and Metabolism* 2001 (August); 86(8):3512–5.

Chattha, Ritu, et al. "Treating the Climacteric Symptoms in Indian Women with an Integrated Approach to Yoga Therapy: A Randomized Control Study." *Menopause.* 2008 Sep–Oct 15(5) 862–70.

Chung, F., et al. "Dose–Response Effects of *Lepidium meyenii* (Maca) Aqueous Extract on Testicular Function and Weight of Different Organs in Adult Rats." *Journal of Ethnopharmacology* 2005; 98(1–2): 143–147.

Clayton, Anita, et al. "Recognition of Depression among Women Presenting with Menopausal Symptoms." *Menopause* 2008 (February): 758-67.

Colbin, Annemarie. *The Book of Whole Meals: A Seasonal Guide to Assembling Balanced Vegetarian Breakfasts, Lunches and Dinners.* Ballantine Books. 1985.

Colbin, Annemarie. *Food and Healing.* Ballantine Books. 1986.

Colbin, Annemarie. *Natural Gourmet.* Ballantine Books. 1991.

Cooper, A., et al. "Systemic Absorption of Progesterone from Progest Cream in Postmenopausal Women." *Lancet* 1998 (April 25):351.

Demers, Laurence et al. "Laboratory Support for the Diagnosis and Monitoring of Thyroid Disease," *The National Academy of Clinical Biochemistry Laboratory Medicine Practice Guidelines*, NACB Publications, 2002.

Dessole, S., et al. "Efficacy of Low-Dose Intravaginal Estriol on Urogenital Aging in Postmenopausal Women." *Menopause* 2004; 11:49–56.

Diaz, Beatriz Lopez, et al. "Endocrine Regulation of the Course of Menopause by Oral Melatonin: First Case Report." *Menopause* 2008; 15(2):388–392.

Dugal, R., et al. "Comparison of Usefulness of Estradiol Vaginal Tablets and Estriol Vagitories for Treatment of Vaginal Atrophy." *Acta Obstetricia et Gynecologica Scandinavica* 2000; 79:293–297.

Eisen, Andrea, et al. "Hormone Therapy and the Risk of Breast Cancer in *BRCA1* Mutation Carriers." *Journal of the National Cancer Institute Advance Access* 2008 (September 23):1361–7.

Elavsky, S., et al. "Physical Activity and Mental Health Outcomes during Menopause: A Randomized Controlled Trial." *Annals of Behavioral Medicine* 2007; 33(2):132–142.

Elkins, Gary, et al. "Randomized Trial of a Hypnosis Intervention for Treatment of Hot Flashes among Breast Cancer Survivors." *Journal of Clinical Oncology* 2008 Nov 1; 26(31):5022–6.

"Estrogen and Progestogen Use in Postmenopausal Women: July 2008 Position Statement of the North American Menopause Society." *Menopause,* 2008;15(4):584–603.

FDA Consumer Health Information. "Bio-Identicals: Sorting Myths from Facts." April 8, 2008. http://www.fda.gov/consumer/updates/bioidenticals040808.html.

"Female Sexual Dysfunction: Evaluation and Treatment." *American Family Physician.* July 1, 2000. http://www.aafp.org/afp/20000701/127.html.

Fox, C. S., et al. "Relations of Thyroid Function to Body Weight: Cross-Sectional and Longitudinal Observations in a Community-based Sample." *Archives of Internal Medicine* 2008; 168(6):587–592.

Freedman, R., et al. "Biochemical and Thermoregulatory Effects of Behavioral Treatment for Menopausal Hot Flashes. *Menopause* 1995; 2(4):211–218.

Freeman, E. W. "Symptomatology of Hot Flashes Mood." Endocrine Society, Endo 2008 poster presentations (S4-1). June 15, 2008

Geller, Stacie, et al. "Botanical and Dietary Supplements for Mood and Anxiety in Menopausal Women." *Menopause* 2007; 14(3):541–549.

Gittleman, Ann Louise. *Before the Change: Taking Charge of Your Perimenopause.* HarperOne. 2003.

Gittleman, Ann Louise. *The Fat Flush Plan.* McGraw-Hill. 2001.

Gittleman, Ann Louise. *Hot Times: How to Eat Well, Live Healthy, and Feel Sexy during the Change.* Avery Publishing Group. 2005.

Gittleman, Ann Louise. *The Gut Flush Plan: The Breakthrough Cleansing Program to Rid Your Body of the Toxins That Make You Sick, Tired, and Bloated.* Avery Publishing Group, 2008.

Gittleman, Ann Louise. *Why Am I Always So Tired?* HarperOne. 1999.

Gold, Ellen B., et al. "Factors Associated with Age at Natural Menopause in a Multiethnic Sample of Midlife Women." *American Journal of Epidemiology* 2001; 153(9):865–874.

Goldstein, Steven R. *The Estrogen Alternative.* Putnam. 1998.

Gonzales, G. F., et al. "Effect of Alcoholic Extract of *Lepidium meyenii* (Maca) on Testicular Function in Male Rats." *Asian Journal of Andrology* 2003; 5(4):349–352.

Gonzales, G. F., et al. "Effect of *Lepidium meyenii* (Maca), a root with Aphrodisiac and Fertility-enhancing Properties, on Serum Reproductive Hormone Levels in Adult Healthy Men." *Journal of Endocrinology* 2003; 176(1):163–168.

Gonzales, G. F., et al. "Effect of *Lepidium meyenii* (Maca) on Sexual Desire and Its Absent Relationship with Serum Testosterone Levels in Adult Healthy Men." *Andrologia* 2002; 34(6):367–372.

Gonzales, G. F., et al. "Red Maca (*Lepidium meyenii*) Reduced Prostate Size in Rats." *Reproductive Biology and Endocrinology* 2005; 3(1):5.

Gould, D. "Uterine Problems: The Menstrual Cycle." *Nursing Standard* 1998; 12(50):38–45.

Grady, Deborah. "Management of Menopausal Symptoms." *New England Journal of Medicine* 2006; 355:2338–2347.

Granberg, S., et al. "Endometrial Sonographic and Histologic Findings in Women with and without Hormonal Replacement Therapy Suffering from Postmenopausal Bleeding. *Maturitas* 1997; 27:35–40.

Greene, Gayle. *Insomniac.* University of California Press. 2008.

Greene, Gayle. "Why Can't Women Sleep?" *Alternet.* July 3, 2008. http://www.alternet.org/story/90001.

Gurgevich, Steven, and Joy Gurgevich. *The Self-Hypnosis Diet: Use the Power of Your Mind to Make Any Diet Work for You/Audio CD.* Sounds True. 2006.

Gurgevich, Steven, and Joy Gurgevich. *The Self-Hypnosis Diet: Use the Power of Your Mind to Reach Your Perfect Weight.* Sounds True. 2007.

Hall, Harriet. "Bioidentical Hormones: Estrogen Is Good. No, It's Bad. No, It's Good." *Eskeptic.* August 15, 2007. http://www.skeptic.com/eskeptic/07-08-15.html.

Hayashi, T., et al. "Estriol (E3) Replacement Improves Endothelial Function and Bone Mineral Density in Very Elderly Women." *Journals of Gerontology. Series A. Biological Sciences and Medical Sciences.* 2000; 55: B183–B190.

Hertoghe, Thierry. *The Hormone Handbook.* International Medical Books. 2006.

Hertoghe, Thierry. *The Hormone Solution: Stay Younger Longer with Natural Hormone and Nutrition Therapies.* Three Rivers Press. 2002.

Hitchcock, C. L., et al. "In Healthy Women Increased Premenstrual Symptoms Present in Ovulatory Cycles Also Occur in Anovulatory Cycles." Endocrine Society, Endo 2008 poster presentations (P2-510). June 16, 2008.

Holland, E. F., et al. "Increase in Bone Mass of Older Postmenopausal Women with Low Mineral Bone Density after One Year of Percutaneous Oestradiol Implants." *British Journal of Obstetrics and Gynaecology* 1995; 102:238–242.

Horsby, P. P., et al. "Cigarette Smoking and Disturbance of Menstrual Function." *Epidemiology* 1998; 9:193–198.

Irvin, J. H., et al. "The Effects of Relaxation Response Training on Menopausal Symptoms." *Journal of Psychosomatic Obstetrics and Gynecology* 1996; 17(4):202–207.

Itoi, H., et al. "Comparison of the Long-Term Effects of Oral Estriol with the Effects of Conjugated Estrogen, 1-Alpha-Hydroxyvitamin D_3 and Calcium Lactate on Vertebral Bone Loss in Early Menopausal Women." *Maturitas* 1997; 28:11–17.

Ivanhoe News Service. "Sexual Chemistry: Diseases and Dysfunction." November 2005. http://www.ivanhoe.com.

Jeffries, William. "Low Dosage Corticoid Therapy." *Archives of Internal Medicine* 1967; 119:265–278.

Jeffries, William. "The Present Status of ACTH, Cortisone, and Related

Steroids in Clinical Medicine." *New England Journal of Medicine* 1955; 253:441–446.

Jeffries, William. *Safe Uses of Cortisone*. Charles C Thomas. 1981.

Kolata, Gina. "Hormones and Cancer: Assessing the Risks." *New York Times*, December 26, 2006.

Krassas, Gerasimos E. "The Male and Female Reproductive System in Hypothyroidism." In Lewis E. Braverman et al. (eds.), *Werner and Ingbar's The Thyroid: A Fundamental and Clinical Text*. Lippincott Williams & Wilkins. 2005:685–723.

Langer, Steven, and James Scheer. *Solved: The Riddle of Illness* (4th ed.). McGraw-Hill. 2006.

Laumann, Edward, et al. "Sexual Dysfunction in the United States: Prevalence and Predictors." *Journal of the American Medical Association* 1999; 281(6):537–44.

Lauria, Joe. "Barbara Seaman: Muckraker for Women's Health." *Women's Enews*. October 17, 2003. http://www.womensenews.org/article.cfm?aid=1566.

LeBlanc, E. S., et al. "Relationship between Estradiol Fluctuations over 24 Hours and Menopausal Symptoms." Endocrine Society, Endo 2008 poster presentations (P2-509). June 16, 2008.

Lee, John, and Virginia Hopkins. *What Your Doctor May Not Tell You about Menopause: The Breakthrough Book on Natural Hormone Balance*. Grand Central Publishing. 2004.

Lee, John, Jesse Hanley, and Virginia Hopkins. *What Your Doctor May Not Tell You About: Premenopause*. Grand Central Publishing. 2005.

Le Guin, Ursula. "The Space Crone." In A. C. Sumerall and D. Taylor (eds.), *Women of the 14th Moon: Writings on Menopause*. The Crossing Press. 1991.

Lemon, H. M., et al. "Inhibition of Radiogenic Mammary Carcinoma in Rats by Estriol or Tamoxifen. *Cancer* 1989; 63:1685–1692.

Lemon, H. M., et al. "Pathophysiologic Considerations in the Treatment of Menopausal Patients with Oestrogens: The Role of Oestriol in the Prevention of Mammary Carcinoma." *Acta Endocrinologica*. Supplementum 1980; 233:17–27.

Lemon, H. M., et al. "Reduced Estriol Excretion in Patients with Breast Cancer Prior to Endocrine Therapy." *Journal of the American Medical Association* 1966; 196:1128–1136.

Leonetti, H. B., J. Landes, J. D. Steinberg, and J. N. Anasti. "Transdermal Progesterone Cream as an Alternative Progestin in Hormone Therapy." *Alternative Therapies in Health and Medicine* 2005; 11:36–38.

Leonetti, H. B., S. Longo, and J. N. Anasti. "Transdermal Progesterone Cream for Vasomotor Symptoms and Postmenopausal Bone Loss." *Obstetrics and Gynecology* 1999; 94(2):225–228.

Leonetti, H. B., K. J. Wilson, and J. N. Anasti. "Topical Progesterone Cream Has an Antiproliferative Effect on Estrogen-stimulated Endometrium." *Fertility and Sterility* 2003; 79(1):221–222.

Lewis, J. E., et al. "A Randomized Controlled Trial of the Effect of Dietary Soy and Flaxseed Muffins on Quality of Life and Hot Flashes during Menopause." *Menopause* 2006; 13(4):631–642.

Liang, Y. L., et al. "Effects of Estrogen and Progesterone on Age-related Changes in Arteries of Postmenopausal Women." *Clinical and Experimental Pharmacology and Physiology.* Aug 24(8):646.

Lippman, M., et al. "Effects of Estrone, Estradiol and Estriol on Hormone-Responsive Human Breast Cancer in Long-Term Tissue Culture." *Cancer Research* 1977; 37:1901–1907.

Lokkegaard, Ellen, et al. "Hormone Therapy and Risk of Myocardial Infarction: A National Register Study." *European Heart Journal* 1993 Nov; 29(21):2660–8.

Lomranz, J. "Attitudes towards Hormone Replacement Therapy among Middle-aged Women and Men." *European Journal of Obstetrics and Gynecology and Reproductive Biology* 2000; 93(2):199–203.

Lopez Diaz, Beatriz, et al. "Endocrine Regulation of the Course of Menopause by Oral Melatonin: First Case Report." *Menopause,* 2008; 15(2):388–392.

Low Dog, Tieraona, et al. "Critical Evaluation of the Safety of *Cimicifuga racemosa* in Menopause Symptom Relief." *Menopause* 2003;10(4):299–313.

Melby, Melissa, et al. "Culture and Symptom Reporting at Menopause." *Human Reproduction Update* 2005;11(5):495–512.

Mercuro, G., et al. "Effects of Acute Administration of Natural Progesterone on Peripheral Vascular Responsiveness in Healthy Postmenopausal Women." *American Journal of Cardiology* 1999; 84(2):214–218.

Michaud, Ellen. "Healing with Your Sixth Sense." *Prevention.* October 2003 issue.

Michel, Joanna, et al. "Symptoms, Attitudes and Treatment Choices Surrounding Menopause among the Q'eqchi Maya of Livingston, Guatemala." *Social Science and Medicine* 2006; 63(3):732–742.

Minaguchi, H., et al. "Effect of Estriol on Bone Loss in Postmenopausal Japanese Women: A Multicenter Prospective Open Study." *Journal of Obstetrics and Gynaecology Research* 1996; 22:259–265.

Montoneri, C., et al. "Effects of Estriol Administration on Human Postmenopausal Endometrium." *Clinical and Experimental Obstetrics and Gynecology* 1987; 14:178–181.

Nagourney, Eric. "Exercise: Increased Physical Activity Aids Menopausal Women." *New York Times*, April 3, 2007.

National Institutes of Health, National Institute of Child Health and Human Development. "Do I Have Premature Ovarian Failure?" U.S. Department of Health and Human Services, 2004. http://www.nichd.nih.gov/publications/pubs/pof/sub3.htm.

Nedrow, Anne, et al. "Complementary and Alternative Therapies for the Management of Menopause-related Symptoms: A Systematic Evidence Review." *Archives of Internal Medicine* 2006 Jul 24; 166(14):1453–66.

Nelson, Lawrence. "Ovarian Insufficiency." *Emedicine*. May 17, 2005. http://www.emedicine.com/med/topic3374.htm.

Newton, Katherine M., et al. "Treatment of Vasomotor Symptoms of Menopause with Black Cohosh, Multibotanicals, Soy, Hormone Therapy, or Placebo: A Randomized Trial." *Annals of Internal Medicine* 2006; 145(112):869–879.

North American Menopause Society. *Early Menopause Guidebook* (6th ed.). North American Menopause Society. 2006.

North American Menopause Society. *Menopause Guidebook* (6th ed.). North American Menopause Society. 2006.

North American Menopause Society. *Menopause Practice: A Clinician's Guide* (3rd ed.). North American Menopause Society. 2007.

North American Menopause Society. "Hormone Products for Postmenopausal Use in the United States and Canada" fact sheet. October 15, 2007.

Nozaki, M., et al. "Usefulness of Estriol for the Treatment of Bone Loss in Postmenopausal Women." *Nippon Sanka Fujinka Gakkai Zasshi* 1996; 48:83–88.

Parker-Pope, Tara. *The Hormone Decision*. Rodale Books. 2007.

Parker-Pope, Tara. "Study Details Women's Risks after Stopping Hormones." *New York Times*, March 5, 2008.

Pierpaoli, Walter (ed.). *Reversal of Aging: Resetting the Pineal Clock*. Wiley-Blackwell. 2006.

Pierpaoli, W., et al. "Effects of Melatonin in Perimenopausal and Menopausal Women: A Randomized and Placebo-Controlled study." *Experimental Gerontology* 2001; 36:297–310.

Pierpaoli, Walter, and William Regelson. *The Melatonin Miracle: Nature's Age-Reversing, Disease-Fighting, Sex-Enhancing Hormone*. Pocket Books. 1996.

Pluchino, N., et al. "One Year Therapy with 10 mg/day DHEA Alone or in Combination with HRT in Postmenopausal Women." Endocrine Society, Endo 2008 poster presentations (P2-511). June 16, 2008.

Power Surge Live. "Exploding the Estrogen Myth: Interview with Barbara Seaman." 2003. http://www.power-surge.com/transcripts/seaman.htm.

Prior, Jerilynn. "For Healthcare Providers: Managing Menorrhagia without Surgery." Centre for Menstrual Cycle and Ovulation Research. December 6, 2007. http://www.cemcor.ubc.ca/help_yourself/articles/managing_menorrhagia.

Prior, Jerilynn. "Natural Help for Hot Flushes." Centre for Menstrual Cycle and Ovulation Research. December 5, 2007. http://www.cemcor.ubc.ca/ask/natural_help_for_hot_flushes.

Prior, Jerilynn. "Perimenopause: The Complex Endocrinology of the Menopausal Transition. *Endocrine Reviews* 1998; 19(4):397–428.

Prior, Jerilynn. "Progesterone as a Bone-trophic Hormone." *Endocrine Reviews* 1990; 11(2):386–398.

Prior, Jerilynn. "Perimenopause Is a Time of 'Endogenous Ovarian Hyperstimulation.'" Centre for Menstrual Cycle and Ovulation Research. December 6, 2007. http://www.cemcor.ubc.ca/help_yourself/articles/perimenopause_endogenous_ovarian_hyperstimulation.

Prior, Jerilynn. "Perimenopause: The Ovary's Frustrating Grand Finale." Centre for Menstrual Cycle and Ovulation Research. December 6, 2007. http://www.cemcor.ubc.ca/help_yourself/articles/perimenopause_ovarys_grand_finale.

Prior, Jerilynn. "Progesterone (Not Estrogen) for Hot Flushes in Perimenopausal and Menopausal Women." Centre for Menstrual Cycle and Ovulation Research. December 5, 2007. http://www.cemcor.ubc.ca/help_yourself/articles/progesterone_hot_flushes.

Prior, Jerilynn. "Very Heavy Menstrual Flow." Centre for Menstrual Cycle and Ovulation Research. December 6, 2007. http://www.cemcor.ubc.ca/help_yourself/articles/very_heavy_menstrual_flow.

Punnonen, R., et al. "The Effect of Oral Estriol Succinate Therapy on the Endometrial Morphology in Postmenopausal Women: The Significance of Fractionation of the Dose." *European Journal of Obstetrics, Gynecology, and Reproductive Biology* 1983; 14:217–224.

Raz, R., et al. "A Controlled Trial of Intravaginal Estriol in Postmenopausal Women with Recurrent Urinary Tract Infections." *New England Journal of Medicine* 1993; 329:753–756.

Red Hot Mamas, "Red Hot Mamas Report: Life Between the Sheets," Winter 2007/2008, http://www.redhotmamas.org/pdf/sex_newsletter.pdf.

Reed, Susan D.,, et al. "Vaginal, Endometrial, and Reproductive Hormone Findings: Randomized, Placebo-Controlled Trial of Black Cohosh, Multibotanical Herbs, and Dietary Soy for Vasomotor Symptoms: The Herbal Alternatives for Menopause (HALT) Study." *Menopause* 2008; 15(1):51–58.

Reiss, Uzzi, and Yfat Reiss Gendell. *The Natural Superwoman: The Scientifically Backed Program for Feeling Great, Looking Younger, and Enjoying Amazing Energy at Any Age.* Avery. 2007.

Rossouw, J. E., et al. "Risks and Benefits of Estrogen Plus Progestin in Healthy Postmenopausal Women: Principal Results from the Women's Health Initiative Randomized Controlled Trial." *Journal of the American Medical Association,* 288(3):321–33.

Savard, Marie. *Apples and Pears: The Body Shape Solution for Weight Loss and Wellness.* Atria Books. 2007.

Savard, Marie. *How to Save Your Own Life: The Eight Steps Only You Can Take to Manage and Control Your Health Care.* Grand Central Publishing. 2000.

Savard, Marie. *The Savard Health Record: A Six-Step System for Managing Your Healthcare.* Time-Life Books. 2000.

Schneider, R., et al. "The Effect of Levothyroxine Therapy on Bone Mineral Density: a Systematic Review of the Literature." *Clinical Endocrinology and Diabetes.* 2003 Dec; 111(8)455–70.

Seaman, Barbara, and Laura Eldridge. *The No-Nonsense Guide to Menopause.* Simon & Schuster. 2008.

Shames, Richard, and Karilee Shames. *Feeling Fat, Fuzzy and Frazzled.* Hudson. 2005.

Shames, Richard, and Karilee Shames. *Thyroid Power: 10 Steps to Total Health,* Collins Living, 2002.

Shapiro, Jerry. "Hair Loss in Women." *New England Journal of Medicine* 2007; 357:1620–1630.

Shea, J. L. "Chinese Women's Symptoms: Relation to Menopause, Age and Related Attitudes." *Climacteric* 2006; 9(1):30–39.

Shifren, Jan L., et al. "A Randomized, Open-Label, Crossover Study Comparing the Effects of Oral versus Transdermal Estrogen Therapy on Serum Androgens, Thyroid Hormones, and Adrenal Hormones in Naturally Menopausal Women." *Menopause* 2007; 14(6):985–994.

Shomon, Mary J. *Living Well with Autoimmune Disease: What Your Doctor Doesn't Tell You . . . That You Need to Know.* HarperResource. 2002.

Shomon, Mary J. *Living Well with Chronic Fatigue Syndrome and Fibromyalgia: What Your Doctor Doesn't Tell You . . . That You Need to Know.* HarperResource. 2004.

Shomon, Mary J. *Living Well with Graves' Disease and Hyperthyroidism:*

What Your Doctor Doesn't Tell You . . . That You Need to Know. Harper-Collins. 2005.

Shomon, Mary J. *Living Well with Hypothyroidism: What Your Doctor Doesn't Tell You . . . That You Need to Know* (2nd ed.). HarperResource. 2005.

Shomon, Mary J. *The Thyroid Diet: Manage Your Metabolism for Lasting Weight Loss.* HarperResource. 2004.

Shomon, Mary J. *The Thyroid Hormone Breakthrough: Overcoming Sexual and Hormonal Problems at Every Age.* HarperResource. 2006.

Sievert, L. L., et al. "Vasomotor Symptoms among Japanese-American and European-American Women Living in Hilo, Hawaii." *Menopause* 2007; 14(2):261–269.

Sowers, M., et al. "Thyroid-Stimulating Hormone (TSH) Concentrations and Menopausal Status in Women at the Mid-life: SWAN." *Clinical Endocrinology* 2003; 58(3):340–347.

"Stealth Tips for Adding Exercise to Your Day—without Going to the Gym" Harvard Health newsletter. August 28, 2008.

Takahashi K, et al. "Efficacy and Safety of Oral Estriol for Managing Postmenopausal Symptoms." *Maturitas* 2000; 34:169–177.

Talk of the Nation. "Can't Sleep? Neither Can 60 Million Other Americans." National Public Radio Interview with Gayle Greene, May 20, 2008.

Tamura, H., et al. "Melatonin Treatment in Peri- and Postmenopausal Women Elevates Serum High-Density Lipoprotein Cholesterol Levels without Influencing Total Cholesterol Levels." *Journal of Pineal Research* 2008; 45:101–105.

Tapp, Teresa, and Barbara Smalley. *Fit and Fabulous in 15 Minutes.* Ballantine Books. 2006.

Taubes, Gary. *Good Calories, Bad Calories.* Knopf. 2007.

Teede, H. J., et al. "A Placebo-Controlled Trial of Long-Term Oral Combined Continuous Hormone Replacement Therapy in Postmenopausal Women: Effects on Arterial Compliance and Endothelial Function. *Clinical Endocrinology* 2001; 55(5):673–682.

Teitelbaum, Jacob. *From Fatigued to Fantastic!* Avery. 2007.

Turgeon, J. "Estrogen and the Brain: Is It All a Matter of Timing?" Endocrine Society, Endo 2008 poster presentations (S4-3). June 15, 2008.

"Understanding the Controversy: Hormone Testing and Bioidentical Hormones." *Menopause.* Oct 11, 2006; http://www.menopause.org/edumaterials/PGO6monograph.pdf.

University of Illinois at Chicago. "Hot Flashes Underreported and Linked to Forgetfulness." Press release. June 17, 2008.

Vakkuri O, et al. "Decrease in Melatonin Precedes Follicle-Stimulating Hormone Increase during Perimenopause." *European Journal of Endocrinology* 1996; 135(2):188–192.

van der Linden, M. C., et al. "The Effect of Estriol on the Cytology of Urethra and Vagina in Postmenopausal Women with Genito-urinary Symptoms. *European Journal of Obstetrics, Gynecology, and Reproductive Biology* 1993; 51:29–33.

Van Voorhis, Bradley, et al. "Anovulation Is Associated with Changes in Menstrual Cycle Timing But Not Heavy Bleeding in the Menopause Transition." *Obstetrics and Gynecology* 2008;112:101–108.

Verduijn, PG. "Late Health Effects of Radiation for Eustachian Tube Dysfunction: Previous Results and Ongoing Study in The Netherlands." *Otolaryngology Head and Neck Surgery.* 1996 Nov; 115(5):417–21.

Vooijs, G. P., et al. "Review of the Endometrial Safety during Intravaginal Treatment with Estriol." *European Journal of Obstetrics, Gynecology, and Reproductive Biology* 1995; 62:101–106.

Wechsler, Toni. *Taking Charge of Your Fertility: The Definitive Guide to Natural Birth Control, Pregnancy Achievement, and Reproductive Health* (rev. ed.). Quill. 2001.

Weiderpass, E., et al. "Low-Potency Oestrogen and Risk of Endometrial Cancer: A Case-Control Study." *Lancet* 1999; 353:1824–1828.

Wenzel, Eberhard, and Gabriella Berger. "Women, Body and Society: Cross-Cultural Differences in Menopause Experiences." Eberhard Wenzel. 2001. http://www.ldb.org/menopaus.htm.

Women's Health Initiative Web site, Department of Health and Human Services, National Institutes of Health, National Heart, Lung, and Blood Institute, http://www.nhlbi.nih.gov/whi.

Wylie-Rosett, Judith. "Menopause, Micronutrients, and Hormone Therapy." *American Journal of Clinical Nutrition* 2005 May 8:1223–1231.

Zhang, W. Y., et al. Efficacy of Minor Analgesics in Primary Dysmenorrhea: A Systematic Review." *British Journal of Obstetrics and Gynaecology* 1998; 105; 780–789.

index